A–Z of Chest Radiology

A–Z of Chest Radiology provides a comprehensive, concise, easily accessible radiological guide to the imaging of acute and chronic chest conditions. Organised in A–Z format by disorder, each entry gives easy access to the key clinical features of a disorder.

An introductory chapter guides the reader in how to review chest X-rays accurately. This is followed by a detailed discussion of over 60 chest disorders, listing appearances, differential diagnoses, clinical features, radiological advice and management. Each disorder is highly illustrated to aid diagnosis; the management advice is concise and practical.

A–Z of Chest Radiology is an invaluable pocket reference for the busy clinician as well as an aid-mémoire for revision in higher exams in both medicine and radiology.

Andrew Planner is a Specialist Registrar in Radiology at John Radcliffe Hospital, Oxford.

Mangerira C. Uthappa is a Consultant Radiologist in the Department of Radiology at Stoke Mandeville Hospital, Buckinghamshire Hospitals NHS Trust.

Rakesh R. Misra is a Consultant Radiologist in the Department of Radiology at Wycombe Hospital, Buckinghamshire Hospitals NHS Trust.

A–Z of Chest Radiology

Andrew Planner, BSc, MB ChB, MRCP, FRCR
Specialist Registrar in Radiology
John Radcliffe Hospital, Oxford

Mangerira C. Uthappa, BSc, MB BS, FRCS, FRCR
Consultant Radiologist, Stoke Mandeville Hospital
Buckinghamshire Hospitals NHS Trust

Rakesh R. Misra, BSc (Hons), FRCS, FRCR
Consultant Radiologist, Wycombe Hospital
Buckinghamshire Hospitals NHS Trust

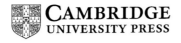
CAMBRIDGE
UNIVERSITY PRESS

CAMBRIDGE UNIVERSITY PRESS
Cambridge, New York, Melbourne, Madrid, Cape Town, Singapore, São Paulo

Cambridge University Press
The Edinburgh Building, Cambridge CB2 8RU, UK

Published in the United States of America by Cambridge University Press, New York

www.cambridge.org
Information on this title: www.cambridge.org/9780521691482

First published 2007

Printed in the United Kingdom at the University Press, Cambridge

A catalogue record for this publication is available from the British Library

ISBN 978-0-521-69148-2 paperback

For my late father, Charles – a brilliant man! **A. C. P.**

Dedicated to my late father Major M. M. Chinnappa for providing support and inspiration. **M. C. U.**

Dedicated to the next generation; my beautiful children, Rohan, Ela and Krishan. **R. R. M.**

CONTENTS

Contents

ABBREVIATIONS

ABC	Airways, breathing and circulation
ABPA	Allergic bronchopulmonary aspergillosis
ACE	Angiotensin converting enzyme
c-ANCA	Cytoplasmic anti neutrophil cytoplasmic antibodies
p-ANCA	Perinuclear anti neutrophil cytoplasmic antibodies
AP	Antero-posterior
ARDS	Adult respiratory distress syndrome
α1-AT	Alpha-1 antitrypsin
AVM	Arteriovenous malformation
BAC	Broncho-alveolar cell carcinoma
BiPAP	Bilevel positive airway pressure
BOOP	Bronchiolitis obliterating organising pneumonia
CCAM	Congenital cystic adenomatoid malformation
CNS	Central nervous system
COP	Cryptogenic organising pneumonia
COPD	Chronic obstructive pulmonary disease
CT	Computed tomography
3D-CT	3-Dimensional computed tomography
CVA	Cerebrovascular accident
CXR	Chest X-ray
DIP	Desquamative interstitial pneumonitis
EAA	Extrinsic allergic alveolitis
Echo	Echocardiography
ENT	Ear, nose and throat
FB	Foreign body
FEV_1	Forced expiratory volume in 1 s
FVC	Forced vital capacity
GI	Gastrointestinal
GOJ	Gastro-oesophageal junction
HD	Hodgkin's disease
HRCT	High-resolution computed tomography
HU	Hounsfield unit
IHD	Ischaemic heart disease
IV	Intravenous
IVC	Inferior vena cava
LAM	Lymphangioleiomyomatosis
LCH	Langerhans' cell histiocytosis
LIP	Lymphocytic interstitial pneumonitis
LV	Left ventricle

M, C & S	Microscopy, culture and sensitivity
MRA	Magnetic resonance angiography
MRI	Magnetic resonance imaging
NBM	Nil by mouth
NF1	Neurofibromatosis type 1
NF2	Neurofibromatosis type 2
NGT	Nasogastric tube
NHL	Non-Hodgkin's lymphoma
NSAID	Non-steroidal Antiinflammatory drug
NSCLC	Non small cell lung cancer
NSIP	Non-specific interstitial pneumonitis
OB	Obliterative bronchiolitis
OGD	Oesophago-gastro duodenoscopy
PA	Postero-anterior
pCO_2	Partial pressure of carbon dioxide
PCP	Pneumocystis pneumonia
PDA	Patent ductus arteriosus
PE	Pulmonary embolus
PEEP	Positive end expiratory pressure ventilation
PET	Positron emission tomography
PMF	Progressive massive fibrosis
pO_2	Partial pressure of oxygen
PPH	Primary pulmonary hypertension
PUO	Pyrexia of unknown origin
RA	Rheumatoid arthritis
RA	Right atrium
RBILD	Respiratory bronchiolitis interstitial lung disease
R-L shunt	Right to left shunt
RTA	Road traffic accident
RV	Right ventricle
S. aureus	Staphylococcus aureus
SCLC	Small cell lung cancer
SOB	Shortness of breath
SVC	Superior vena cava
T_1	T_1 weighted magnetic resonance imaging
T_2	T_2 weighted magnetic resonance imaging
TB	Tuberculosis
TIA	Transient ischaemic attack
TOE	Trans-oesophageal echocardiography
UIP	Usual interstitial pneumonitis
US	Ultrasound
$\dot{V}/\dot{Q}$	Ventilation/perfusion scan
VSD	Ventricular septal defect

When interpreting a CXR it is important to make an assessment of whether the x-ray is of diagnostic quality. In order to facilitate this, first pay attention to two radiographic parameters prior to checking for pathology; namely the *quality* of the film and *patient-dependent factors*. A suboptimal x-ray can mask or even mimic underlying disease.

Quality assessment

Is the film correctly labelled?

This may seem like an obvious statement to make. However, errors do occur and those relating to labelling of the radiograph are the most common.

What to check for?
- Does the x-ray belong to the correct patient? Check the patient's name on the film.
- Have the left and right side markers been labelled correctly, or does the patient really have dextrocardia?
- Lastly has the projection of the radiograph (PA vs. AP) been documented?

Assessment of exposure quality

Is the film penetrated enough?

- On a high quality radiograph, the vertebral bodies should just be visible through the heart.
- If the vertebral bodies are not visible, then an insufficient number of x-ray photons have passed through the patient to reach the x-ray film. As a result the film will look 'whiter' leading to potential 'overcalling' of pathology.
- Similarly, if the film appears too 'black', then too many photons have resulted in overexposure of the x-ray film. This 'blackness' results in pathology being less conspicuous and may lead to 'undercalling'.

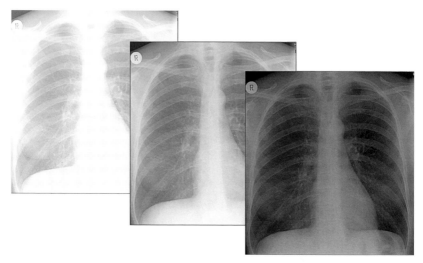

The effect of varied exposure on the quality of the final image.

Is the film PA or AP

- Most CXRs are taken in a PA position; that is, the patient stands in front of the x-ray film cassette with their chest against the cassette and their back to the radiographer. The x-ray beam passes through the patient from back to front (i.e. PA) onto the film. The heart and mediastinum are thus closest to the film and therefore not magnified.
- When an x-ray is taken in an AP position, such as when the patient is unwell in bed, the heart and mediastinum are distant from the cassette and are therefore subject to x-ray magnification. As a result it is very difficult to make an accurate assessment of the cardiomediastinal contour on an AP film.

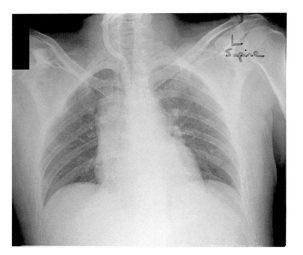

The cardiomediastinal contour is significantly magnified on this AP film. This needs to be appreciated and not overcalled.

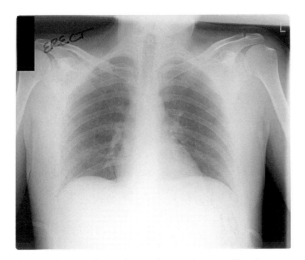

On the PA film, taken only an hour later, the mediastinum appears normal.

Patient-dependent factors

Assessment of patient rotation

- Identifying patient rotation is important. Patient rotation may result in the normal thoracic anatomy becoming distorted; cardiomediastinal structures, lung parenchyma and the bones and soft tissues may all

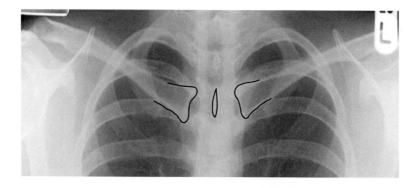

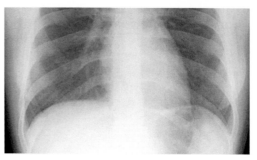

A well centred x-ray. Medial ends of clavicles are equidistant from the spinous process.

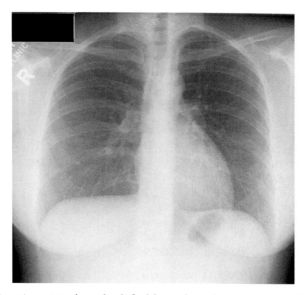

This patient is rotated to the left. Note the spinous process is close to the right clavicle and the left lung is 'blacker' than the right, due to the rotation.

appear more, or less, conspicuous. To the uninitiated, failure to appreciate this could easily lead to 'overcalling' pathology.

- On a high-quality CXR, the medial ends of both clavicles should be equidistant from the spinous process of the vertebral body projected between the clavicles. If this is not the case then the patient is rotated, either to the left or to the right.
- If there is rotation, the side to which the patient is rotated is assessed by comparing the densities of the two hemi-thoraces. *The increase in blackness of one hemi-thorax is always on the side to which the patient is rotated, irrespective of whether the CXR has been taken PA or AP.*

Assessment of adequacy of inspiratory effort

Ensuring the patient has made an adequate inspiratory effort is important in the initial assessment of the CXR.

- Assessment of inspiratory adequacy is a simple process.
- It is ascertained by counting either the number of visible anterior or posterior ribs.
- If six complete anterior or ten posterior ribs are visible then the patient has taken an adequate inspiratory effort.
- Conversely, fewer than six anterior ribs implies a poor inspiratory effort and more than six anterior ribs implies hyper-expanded lungs.

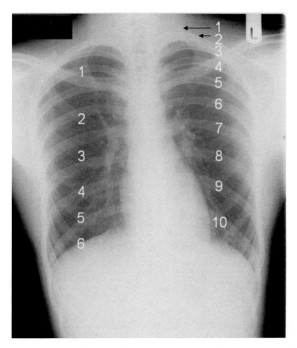

Six complete anterior ribs (and ten posterior ribs) are clearly visible.

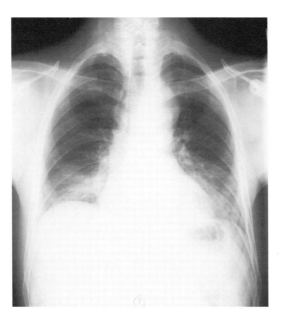

An example of poor inspiratory effort. Only four complete anterior ribs are visible. This results in several spurious findings: cardiomegaly, a mass at the aortic arch and patchy opacification in both lower zones.

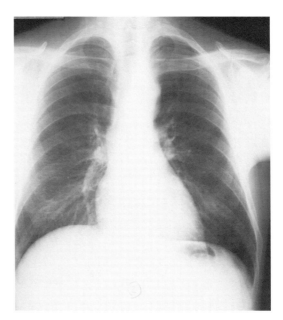

Same patient following an adequate inspiratory effort. The CXR now appears normal.

- If a poor inspiratory effort is made or if the CXR is taken in expiration, then several potentially spurious findings can result:
  - apparent cardiomegaly
  - apparent hilar abnormalities
  - apparent mediastinal contour abnormalities
  - the lung parenchyma tends to appear of increased density, i.e. 'white lung'.
- Needless to say any of these factors can lead to CXR misinterpretation.

Review of important anatomy

Heart and mediastinum

Assessment of heart size

- The cardiothoracic ratio should be less than 0.5.
- i.e. $A/B < 0.5$.
- A cardiothoracic ratio of greater than 0.5 (in a good quality film) suggests cardiomegaly.

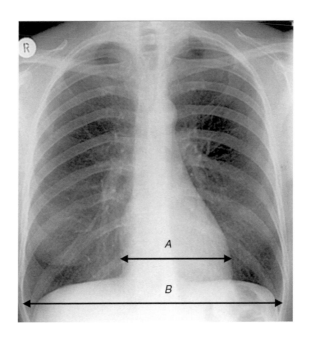

Assessment of cardiomediastinal contour

- **Right side:**
  - SVC
  - RA
- **Anterior aspect:**
  - RV
- **Cardiac apex:**
  - LV
- **Left side:**
  - LV
  - Left atrial appendage
  - Pulmonary trunk
  - Aortic arch.

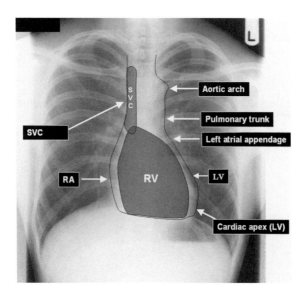

Assessment of hilar regions

- Both hilar should be concave. This results from the superior pulmonary vein crossing the lower lobe pulmonary artery. The point of intersection is known as the *hilar point (**HP**)*.
- Both hilar should be of similar density.
- The left hilum is usually superior to the right by up to 1 cm.

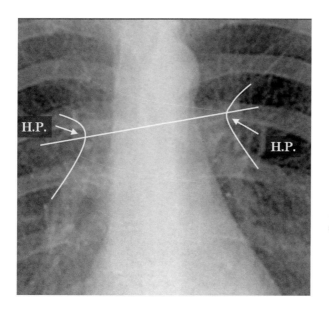

Assessment of the trachea

- The trachea is placed usually just to the right of the midline, but can be pathologically pushed or pulled to either side, providing indirect support for an underlying abnormality.
- The right wall of the trachea should be clearly seen as the so-called right para-tracheal stripe.

- The para-tracheal stripe is visible by virtue of the silhouette sign: air within the tracheal lumen and adjacent right lung apex outline the soft-tissue-density tracheal wall.
- Loss or thickening of the para-tracheal stripe intimates adjacent pathology.
- The trachea is shown in its normal position, just to the right of centre. The right para-tracheal stripe is clearly seen.

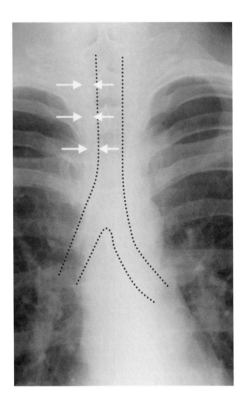

Evaluation of mediastinal compartments

It is useful to consider the contents of the mediastinum as belonging to three compartments:

- *Anterior mediastinum*: anterior to the pericardium and trachea.
- *Middle mediastinum*: between the anterior and posterior mediastinum.
- *Posterior mediastinum*: posterior to the pericardial surface.

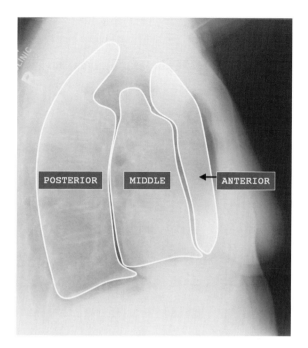

Lungs and pleura

Lobar anatomy

There are three lobes in the right lung and two in the left. The left lobe also contains the lingula; a functionally separate 'lobe', but anatomically part of the upper lobe.

Right lung

- Upper lobe
- Middle lobe
- Lower lobe.

Left lung

- Upper lobe; this contains the lingula
- Lower lobe.

Pleural anatomy

There are two layers of pleura: the parietal pleura and the visceral pleura.

- The parietal pleura lines the thoracic cage and the visceral pleura surrounds the lung.
- Both of these layers come together to form reflections which separate the individual lobes. These pleural reflections are known as *fissures*.
- On the right there is an oblique and horizontal fissure; the right upper

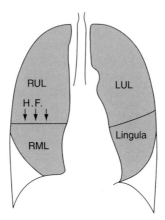

Lobar and pleural anatomy – frontal view.

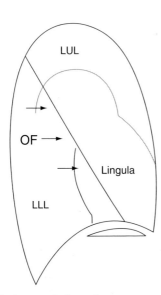

Lobar and pleural anatomy – left lateral view.

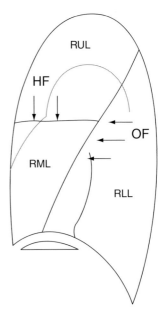

Lobar and pleural anatomy – right lateral view.

lobe sits above the horizontal fissure (HF), the right lower lobe behind the oblique fissure (OF) and the middle lobe between the two.
- On the left, an oblique fissure separates the upper and lower lobes.

Diaphragms

Assessment of the diaphragms

- Carefully examine each diaphragm. The highest point of the right diaphragm is usually 1–1.5 cm higher than that of the left. Each costo-phrenic angle should be sharply outlined. The outlines of both

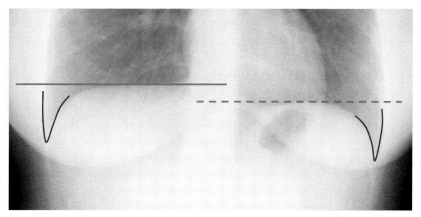

The right hemidiaphragm is 'higher' than the left. Both costophrenic angles are sharply outlined.

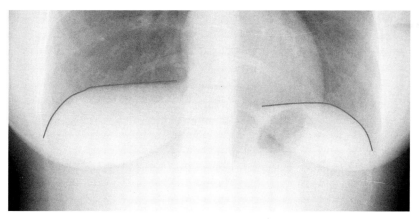

The outlines of both hemidiaphragms should be clearly visible.

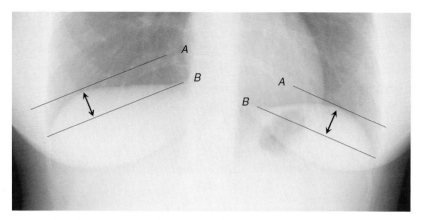

Assess for diaphragmatic flattening. The distance between *A* and *B* should be at least 1.5 cm.

hemidiaphragms should be sharp and clearly visible along their entire length (except the medial most aspect of the left hemidiaphragm).
- The 'curvature' of both hemidiaphragms should be assessed to identify diaphragmatic flattening. The highest point of a hemidiaphragm should be at least 1.5 cm above a line drawn from the cardiophrenic to the costophrenic angle.

Bones and soft tissues

Assessment of bones and soft tissues

This is an area often overlooked. When assessing a CXR, there is a tendency to routinely look at the 'heart and lungs', and skirt over the bones and soft tissues.

It is important to scrutinise every rib (from the anterior to posterior), the clavicles, vertebrae and the shoulder joints (if they are on the film). Similarly, look carefully at the soft tissues for asymmetry; a typical finding in cases following mastectomy. It can be surprisingly difficult to 'see' objects that are missing. If the 'bones and soft tissues' are not given their due consideration then vital information may not be appreciated.

After scrutinising the bones and soft tissues, remember to look for pathology in the 'hidden areas'.
- The lung apices
- Look 'behind' the heart
- Under the diaphragms.

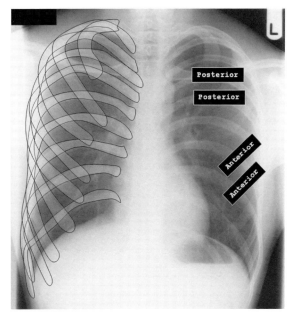

Remember to scrutinise every rib, (from the anterior to posterior), the clavicles vetebrae and the shoulders.

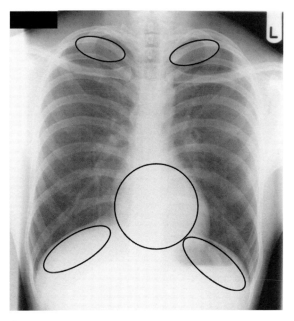

The 'hidden' areas.

I

A brief look at the lateral CXR

Important anatomy relating to the lateral CXR

Key points

- There should be a decrease in density from superior to inferior in the posterior mediastinum.
- The retrosternal airspace should be of the same density as the retro-cardiac airspace.

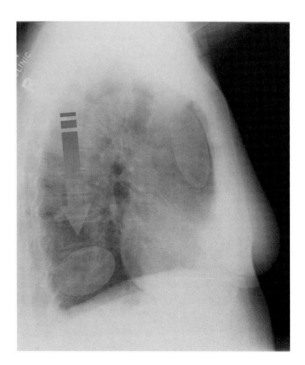

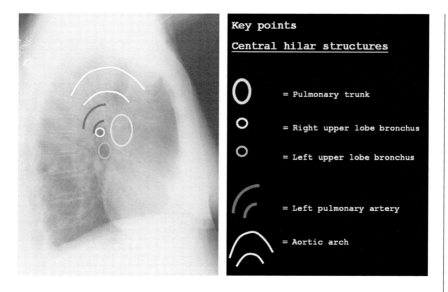

Key points

Central hilar structures

O	= Pulmonary trunk
o	= Right upper lobe bronchus
o	= Left upper lobe bronchus
((	= Left pulmonary artery
⌒	= Aortic arch

Diaphragms

The right hemidiaphragm is usually 'higher' than the left. The outline of the right can be seen extending from the posterior to anterior chest wall. The outline of the left hemidiaphragm stops at the posterior heart border. Air in the gastric fundus is seen below the left hemidiaphragm.

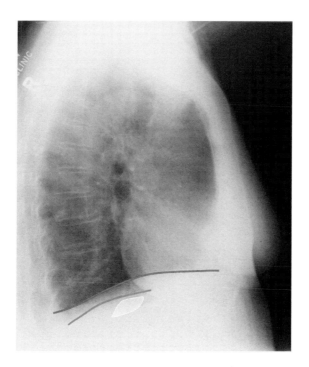

Understanding the silhouette sign

The silhouette sign, first described by Felson in 1950, is a means of detecting and localising abnormalities within the chest.

In order for any object to appear radiographically distinct on a CXR, it must be of a different radiographic density to that of an adjacent structure. Broadly speaking only four different radiographic densities are detectable on a plain radiograph: air, fat, soft tissue and bone (i.e. calcium). If two soft tissue densities lie adjacent to each other, they will not be visible separately (e.g. the left and right ventricles). If however two such densities are separated by air, the boundaries of both will be seen. The silhouette sign has applications elsewhere in the body too; gas is outlined within bowel lumen separate from soft tissue bowel wall, renal outlines are visible due to the presence of perinephric fat between the kidneys and surrounding soft tissues.

The silhouette sign has two uses:

- It can localise abnormalities on a frontal CXR without the aid of a lateral view. For example, if a mass lies adjacent to, and obliterates the outline of, the aortic arch, then the mass lies posteriorly against the arch (which represents the posteriorly placed arch and descending aorta). If the outline of the arch and of the mass are seen separately, then the mass lies anteriorly.

- The loss of the outline of the hemidiaphragm, heart border or other structures suggests that there is soft tissue shadowing adjacent to these, such as lung consolidation. *(See Section 2 for various examples of lung consolidation)*.

A–Z CHEST RADIOLOGY

Abscess

Characteristics

- Cavitating infective consolidation.
- Single or multiple lesions.
- Bacterial (*Staphylococcus aureus*, *Klebsiella*, *Proteus*, *Pseudomonas*, TB and anaerobes) or fungal pathogens are the most common causative organisms.
- 'Primary' lung abscess – large solitary abscess without underlying lung disease is usually due to anaerobic bacteria.
- Associated with aspiration and/or impaired local or systemic immune response (elderly, epileptics, diabetics, alcoholics and the immunosuppressed).

Clinical features

- There is often a predisposing risk factor, e.g. antecedent history of aspiration or symptoms developing in an immunocompromised patient.
- Cough with purulent sputum.
- Swinging pyrexia.
- Consider in chest infections that fail to respond to antibiotics.
- It can run an indolent course with persistent and sometimes mild symptoms. These are associated with weight loss and anorexia mimicking pulmonary neoplastic disease or TB infection.

Radiological features

- Most commonly occur in the apicoposterior aspect of the upper lobes or the apical segment of the lower lobe.
- **CXR** may be normal in the first 72 h.
- **CXR** – a cavitating essentially spherical area of consolidation usually >2 cm in diameter, but can measure up to 12 cm. There is usually an air–fluid level present.
- Characteristically the dimensions of the abscess are approximately equal when measured in the frontal and lateral projections.
- **CT** is important in characterising the lesion and discriminating from other differential lesions. The abscess wall is thick and irregular and may contain locules of free gas. Abscesses abutting the pleura form acute angles. There is no compression of the surrounding lung. The abscess does not cross fissures. It is important to make sure no direct communication with the bronchial tree is present (bronchopleural fistula).

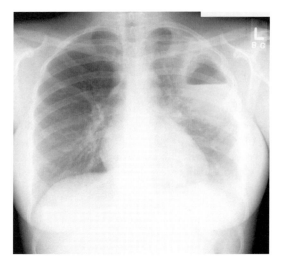

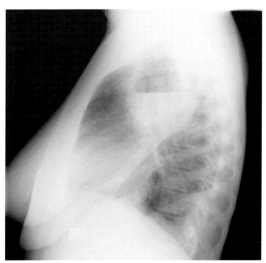

Lung abscess – frontal and lateral views. Cavitating lung abscess in the left upper zone.

Differential diagnosis

- **Bronchopleural fistula** – direct communication with bronchial tree. Enhancing split pleural layers on CT.
- **Empyema** - enhancing split pleural layers, forming obtuse margins with the lung on CT.
- **Primary or secondary lung neoplasms** (e.g. squamous cell carcinomas) – these lesions can run a slow indolent course. Failure to respond to antibiotic therapy should alert the clinician to the diagnosis.
- **TB** (usually reactivation) – again suspected following slow response to treatment. Other findings on the CT may support old tuberculous infection such as lymph node and/or lung calcification. Lymphadenopathy, although uncommon, may be present on the CT scans in patients with lung abscesses. It is therefore not a discriminating tool for differentiating neoplasms or TB infection.

Management

- Sputum – M, C & S.
- Protracted course of antibiotics is usually a sufficient treatment regime.
- Physiotherapy may be helpful.
- Occasionally percutaneous drainage may be required.
- Lastly, some lesions failing to respond to treatment and demonstrating soft tissue growth or associated with systemic upset (e.g. weight loss) may need biopsy. This is done to exclude underlying neoplasm (e.g. squamous cell carcinoma).

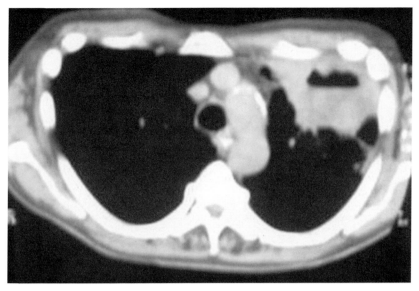

Lung abscess – CT (different patient). CT clearly defines the cavitating abscess in the left upper lobe.

Achalasia

Characteristics

- Achalasia or megaoesophagus is characterised by failure of organised peristalsis and relaxation of the lower oesophageal sphincter.
- Primary or idiopathic achalasia is due to degeneration of Auerbach's myenteric plexus.
- Rarely associated with infections, e.g. Chagas' disease (*Trypanosoma cruzi*) present in South American countries.
- Secondary or pseudoachalasia occurs due to malignant infiltration destroying the myenteric plexus from a fundal carcinoma or lymphoma.
- Oesophageal carcinoma occurs in 2–7% of patients with long-standing achalasia.

Clinical features

- Primarily a disease of early onset – aged 20–40 years.
- Long slow history of dysphagia, particularly to liquids.
- The dysphagia is posturally related. Swallowing improves in the upright position compared to lying prone. The increased hydrostatic forces allow transient opening of the lower oesophageal sphincter.
- Weight loss occurs in up to 90%.
- There is an increased risk of aspiration. Patients can present with chest infections or occult lung abscesses.
- Malignant transformation rarely occurs in long-standing cases and should be suspected with changes in symptoms, e.g. when painful dysphagia, anaemia or continued weight loss develop.

Radiological features

- **CXR** – an air-fluid level within the oesophagus may be present projected in the midline, usually in a retrosternal location, but can occur in the neck. Right convex opacity projected behind the right heart border, occasionally a left convex opacity can be demonstrated. Mottled food residue may be projected in the midline behind the sternum. Accompanying aspiration with patchy consolidation or abscess formation is demonstrated in the apical segment of the lower lobes and/or the apicoposterior segments of the upper lobe.
- **Barium swallow** – a dilated oesophagus beginning in the upper one-third. Absent primary peristalsis. Erratic tertiary contractions. 'Bird beak' smooth tapering at the gastro-oesophageal junction (GOJ) with delayed sudden opening at the GOJ. Numerous tertiary contractions can be present in a non-dilated early oesophageal achalasia (vigorous achalasia).

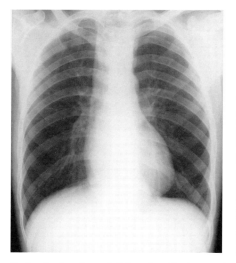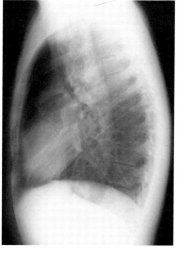

Achalasia. An additional soft tissue density line is seen parallel to the right mediastinal contour. The gastric fundus bubble is absent. On the lateral view, the entire oesophagus is dilated and is of increased density due to contained debris.

Differential diagnosis

- The key differential lies with **malignant pseudoachalasia**. This condition occurs in an older age group (>50) with more rapid onset of symptoms (<6 months). Clinical suspicion should merit an OGD ± a CT scan to look closely for neoplastic change, particularly submucosal or extramural disease.
- **Diffuse oesophageal spasm** can produce similar clinical symptoms. Barium swallow and oesophageal manometry help discriminate this condition from achalasia.

Management

- Diagnosis includes a barium swallow and pressure measurements from oesophageal manometry.
- Oesophageal dilatation is the standard form of treatment and repeated therapies may be necessary.
- Botulinum toxin injection can be effective, but has a short-lived action (<6 months).
- Surveillance for oesophageal carcinoma should be considered.
- Surgical intervention: laparoscopic Heller's cardiomyotomy.

Alveolar microlithiasis

Characteristics

- Very rare disease of unknown aetiology characterised by multiple tiny calculi deposited throughout the alveoli.
- 50% familial tendency.
- Equal sex incidence (M = F).
- Often asymptomatic.
- Peak incidence between ages 30 and 50 years, but probably starts earlier in life.

Clinical features

- Majority have mild symptoms or are asymptomatic (70%).
- Disease progression is variable.
- Exertional dyspnoea is the commonest symptom and the majority of patients remain clinically stable throughout life following the onset of symptoms.
- Cyanosis and clubbing can occur. A minority develop pulmonary fibrosis and subsequent cor pulmonale.
- Normal serum calcium and phosphorus.

Radiological features

- **CXR** – multiple dense very fine sand-like micronodulations (<1 mm). The changes are diffuse and present throughout both lungs. Fibrosis can occur with further changes, including bullae most marked in the lung apices. Chronic cases may be associated with enlargement of the pulmonary arteries in keeping with secondary pulmonary hypertension.
- **Bone scan** – avid uptake of tracer throughout the lungs.

Differential diagnosis

- The main differential diagnosis lies between multiple healed calcified granulomata, particularly following a viral infection and inorganic pneumoconiosis, e.g. heavy metal inhalation. In practice the size of the nodules in these lesions coupled with the antecedent history should alert the clinician to the correct diagnosis.

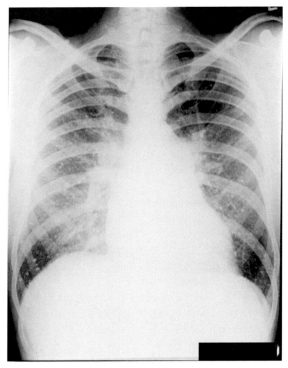

Alveolar microlithiasis. Multiple tiny nodules of high density scattered throughout both lungs.

Management

- No specific therapeutic options. Follow-up in symptomatic patients with assessment of pulmonary function in those who develop fibrosis and pulmonary insufficiency.
- No advantage to family screening in identified cases.

II

Aneurysm of the pulmonary artery

Characteristics

- Permanent dilatation of the main and/or segmental pulmonary arterial branches which can be congenital or acquired.
- **Congenital** – rare condition seen in adolescent females with dilatation of the main pulmonary artery. Patients are usually asymptomatic with only a soft ejection systolic murmur detectable. No significant complications. The diagnosis is made after excluding other acquired conditions.
- **Acquired**
  - Infections (e.g. TB, known as Rasmussen aneurysm, where there is mycotic inflammatory necrosis causing dilatation of the arterial wall).
  - Collagen vascular disorders (e.g. Marfan's syndrome).
  - Inflammatory (e.g. Takayasu's arteritis).
  - Behçet's disease. Segmental artery dilatation is a feature of Hughes–Stovin syndrome.
  - Post trauma – blunt (RTA), or direct (following arterial instrumentation).
  - Post stenotic dilatation in pulmonary valvular stenosis.
  - Thromboembolic disease.
  - Associated with primary bronchial neoplasm.

Clinical features

- Clinical presentation depends on the underlying cause and location of the aneurysm.
- Congenital lesions are uncommon and asymptomatic.
- Acquired lesion – most commonly present with haemoptysis. Rupture may complicate the clinical picture and is frequently fatal.
- In many cases diagnosis is incidental following investigations for the underlying primary disease.

Radiological features

- **CXR** – isolated main pulmonary artery dilatation in the aortopulmonary window with normal lungs is a rare radiological finding. More commonly the aneurysm lies within an ill-defined area of consolidation and is difficult to fully appreciate.
- **Contrast-enhanced CT** scanning allows clearer appreciation of the size, location and extent of the arterial aneurysm(s).
- **CT** also allows for further assessment of the underlying cause. An increasing focal lung mass raises the possibility of aneurysm. Lack of an arterial wall and a history of trauma support the diagnosis of a false aneurysm of the pulmonary artery.

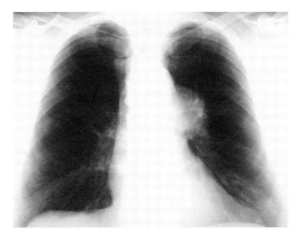

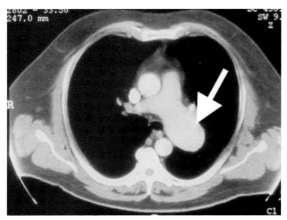

Pulmonary artery aneurysm. Left hilar mass which is of similar density to the right hilum. Note that vessels can be seen through the mass. CT confirms the diagnosis (arrow).

Differential diagnosis

- The main differential lies within the varying underlying causes listed above.

Management

- Management is dependent on identifying the abnormalities, correlating with the clinical history, and excluding the various different conditions.
- Sputum culture, echocardiography, cardiac catheterisation and arterial wall biopsy may all play a role in the diagnostic pathway.
- Treatment options are targeted first at the correct management of the cause.
- Surgical repair of the aneurysm and the use of endovascular stent grafts are rarely used strategies, but potentially offer definitive treatment.

Aortic arch aneurysm

Characteristics

- Permanent localised dilatation of the thoracic aorta. The average diameter of the normal thoracic aorta is <4.5 cm. This is the commonest mediastinal vascular abnormality. Most are fusiform dilatations (some are saccular), associated with degenerative atherosclerosis with a mean age at diagnosis of 65.
- Dissecting aortic aneurysms or intramural haematomas are a specific form of thoracic aneurysm. Again, associated with hypertension and degenerative atherosclerosis, a split in the aortic wall allows blood to track between the intimal and adventitial layers of the aorta. They can occur following trauma. This can produce widening of the aorta and a very high risk of rupture. Slow flow in the false lumen can result in ischaemia and infarction to end organs supplied by the thoracic and ultimately the abdominal aorta. It can be graded by the Stanford classification into **type A** (ascending aorta and arch − 2/3) and **type B** descending aorta distal to major vessels (1/3).
- Other rarer causes include congenital causes, infection (mycotic aneurysms, e.g. bacteria or syphilis), connective tissue disorders (e.g. cystic medial necrosis in Marfan's syndrome), inflammatory diseases (e.g. Takayasu's) and dilatation post aortic valvular stenosis. These occur in a younger age group.
- The size of the aneurysm increases with age.
- The risk of rupture increases with aneurysm size.

Clinical features

- This is commonly found incidentally on routine CXRs in asymptomatic patients.
- The patients may present with substernal, back and/or shoulder pains which can often be severe.
- Rarely patients may present with stridor, hoarse voice or dysphagia from the aneurysm compressing local mediastinal structures.
- Aortic dissection is associated with aortic regurgitation and cardiac failure, heart murmurs and differential blood pressure measurements in the arms. In addition dissecting aneurysms can produce ischaemia and infarction to end organs (e.g. stroke, renal failure, ischaemic bowel).
- Rupture of the aneurysm is almost always fatal with patients presenting with collapse and hypotension from hypovolaemic shock.

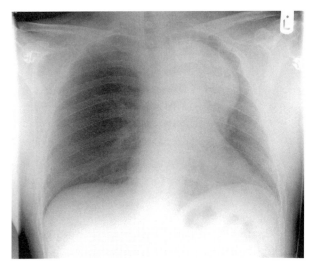

Aortic arch aneurysm.

Radiological features

- **CXR** – a soft tissue mediastinal mass in the region of the aorta, measuring 4–10 cm. Wide tortuous aorta >4.5 cm. Curvilinear calcifications outlining the aortic wall. Left pleural effusions, left apical cap or left lower lobe collapse.
- **CT** – above findings ± extensive mural thrombus present within the aortic wall. In early aortic dissections the aortic wall may be thickened and of slightly increased attenuation. A dissection flap may be demonstrated with a double channel to the aorta. High attenuation lies within the false lumen, which is usually present in the superior aspect of the aortic arch. Contrast-enhanced CT demonstrates the differential flow within the two or more lumens. There may also be evidence of a haemopericardium with retrograde dissection back to the heart.
- **MRI** – contrast-enhanced MRA is a very good alternative to characterising the site and extent of aortic aneurysm, particularly dissecting aneurysms.
- **Transoesophageal echocardiography** – very sensitive in characterising aortic aneurysms and in particular the cardiac involvement in dissecting aneurysms.
- **Angiography** – the true and false lumens demonstrated may be of normal, reduced or enlarged calibre.
- **Rupture** may be associated with high attenuation fluid in the mediastinum and pleural space.

Differential diagnosis

- The differential diagnosis, other than the different types of aortic aneurysm already described, is **chronic aortic pseudoaneurysm**. This occurs in 2.5% of patients who survive the initial trauma of acute aortic transection. There is focal aortic dilatation with disruption of the aortic wall. Blood is contained by adventia and connective tissue only. The pseudoaneurysm increases in size with time and is at risk of rupture.

Management

- Aneurysm repair is considered in all patients when the aneurysmal size increases beyond 6 cm.
- Both surgical and endovascular stent grafting are successful treatment options.
- Surgical mortality is as high as 10%.
- Control of risk factors such as hypertension.
- Surveillance of aneurysms >5 cm.
- Dissecting aneurysms are a surgical emergency. ABC first line, then assessment and grading of the dissection. In particular 3D CT reformats are very helpful for completely assessing the extent and branch artery involvement. Early surgery considered in type A dissections.
- Non-surgical survival rates are lower than 10%.

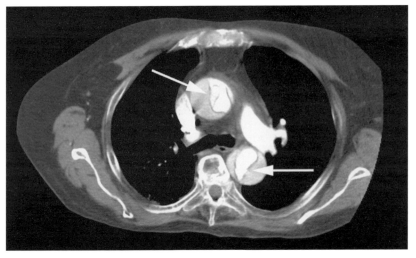

Type A aortic dissection. Dissection 'flaps' can be seen in both the ascending and descending aorta (arrows).

Aortic rupture

Characteristics

- Blood leakage through the aortic wall.
- **Spontaneous rupture**. Hypertension and atherosclerosis predispose to rupture. There may be an underlying aneurysm present, but rupture can occur with no preformed aneurysm.
- **Traumatic rupture** or transection following blunt trauma. Follows deceleration injury (RTA). Over 80% die before arrival at hospital. The weakest point, where rupture is likely to occur, is at the aortic isthmus, which is just distal to the origin of the left subclavian artery.
- The rupture may be revealed or concealed.

Clinical features

- There is often an antecedent history of a known aneurysm or appropriate trauma (e.g. RTA).
- Patients may be asymptomatic particularly if the rupture is small and intramural.
- Most cases present with severe substernal pain radiating through to the back. Patients may be breathless, hypotensive, tachycardic or moribund.

Radiological features

- **CXR** – look for widening of the mediastinum on CXRs. It is very rare to see aortic rupture in a patient with a normal CXR. Other features on the CXR include loss of the aortic contour, focal dilatation of the aorta and a left apical cap (blood tracking up the mediastinal pleural space). Signs of chest trauma – rib fractures (1st and 2nd), haemopneumothorax and downward displacement of a bronchus.
- **Unenhanced CT** – may show crescentic high attenuation within a thickened aortic wall only (intramural haematoma, at risk of imminent dissection or rupture). Rupture is associated with extensive mediastinal blood. A pseudoaneurysm may be present. There may be injuries to major branching vessels from the aorta.
- **Angiography** or **transoesophageal echocardiography** – may be helpful to confirm small intimal tears of the aortic wall. However, contrast-enhanced **MRA** is a sensitive alternative investigation to standard invasive angiography.

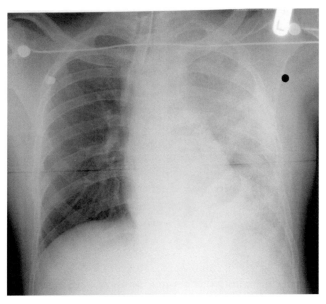

Aortic rupture. The outline of the aortic arch is ill-defined and there is tracheal deviation to the right. Generalised increase in density of the left hemithorax – secondary to haemorrhage. Note additional injuries: rib fractures and diaphragmatic rupture.

Differential diagnosis

- The differential diagnosis for a widened mediastinum on a frontal CXR includes lymphadenopathy, tumours and simple aneurysms. Further assessment, usually with urgent CT imaging, may be required in the first instance if there is any suspicion of thoracic aortic injury.

Management

- ABC – this is a surgical emergency.
- Appropriate imaging and full characterisation of the aortic rupture and, in cases of trauma, other accompanying injuries.
- Early surgical repair. In cases that are considered a high operative risk, patients are considered for aortic stent grafting.
- In patients who survive there is a long-term small risk of chronic pseudoaneurysm formation.

Asbestos plaques

Characteristics

- Asbestos-related pleural plaques represent focal areas of fibrotic response in the visceral pleura to previous exposure to inhaled asbestos fibres at least 8–10 years before. Classically, they calcify (approximately 50%). Both the presence of plaques and their calcification increase with time. They spare the costophrenic angles and lung apices. In their own right they have no malignant potential; however, in some patients, asbestos exposure can lead to pulmonary fibrosis, lung cancer and mesothelioma.

Clinical features

- Asbestos plaques are asymptomatic. Any chest symptoms should alert the clinician to the potential complications of asbestos exposure.

Radiological features

- **CXR** – focal areas of pleural thickening (<1 cm). They are usually bilateral and may be multiple. Plaques are more visible when they calcify and calcified plaques have a thicker peripheral edge than central portion. When they are seen en-face they have an irregular 'holly leaf' appearance. Non-calcified plaques seen en-face can give a patchy density to the lungs. There should be no lymphadenopathy.
- They are associated with rounded atelectasis or pseudotumours. On the **CXR** these look like peripherally based round nodules mimicking lung neoplasms. On **CT** imaging they demonstrate a rounded area of lung abutting an area of pleural thickening, with a swirl of vessels (tail) leading to the peripheral-based lesion. They are completely benign and should be recognised to avoid further invasive investigations.
- Occasionally the pleural thickening can be diffuse, restricting lung function and mimicking mesothelioma.

Differential diagnosis

- There are few conditions which have a similar appearance.
- Previous history of TB or haemorrhagic pleural effusions can give a similar picture (more often unilateral).
- Exposure to amiodarone and a very rare condition of idiopathic pleural fibrosis can also produce these findings.

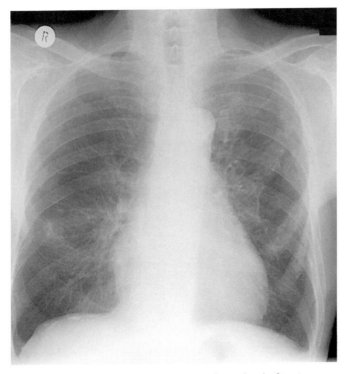

Asbestos plaques. Right diaphragmatic pleural calcification seen. Additional ill-defined pleural calcification also present in the left mid zone.

Management

- No active management.
- Need to exclude complications of asbestos exposure with a supportive clinical history and possibly further imaging (CT scan).
- Consider follow-up, particularly if chest symptoms persist and the patient is a smoker. Pulmonary asbestosis (fibrosis secondary to asbestos exposure) increases the risk of lung cancer 40-fold if the patient is also a smoker.
- Consideration for industrial financial compensation.

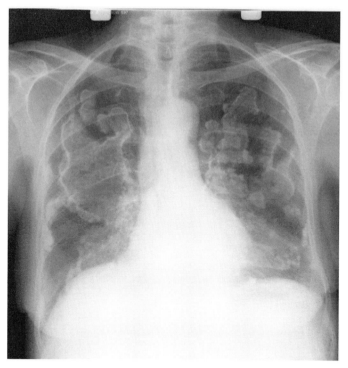

Asbestos plaques. Extensive calcified pleural plaques are seen in both lungs.

Asthma

Characteristics

- Asthma is characterised by a triad of airway inflammation, reversible airway obstruction, and hyper-reactivity of the airways to a variety of stimuli.
- Functionally the disease is characterised by wide variations, over short periods of time, in resistance to air flow in intrapulmonary airways. This increase in airway resistance is reversible, particularly with bronchodilators.
- Intrinsic asthma – no definite precipitating cause. Young and middle-age onset.
- Extrinsic or atopic asthma – immediate type 1 hypersensitivity reaction to specific antigen or allergen (e.g. pollens or chemicals). Removal of the stimulus produces a clinical improvement.

Clinical features

- Attacks of breathlessness, chest tightness and wheeze. Often severe and requiring ventilatory support.
- Occasionally, mild symptoms such as a persistent cough predominate.
- The patient is hypoxic with low pO_2 and usually a low pCO_2. A high pCO_2 is a sinister sign heralding severe fatigue and respiratory failure.
- There is reduced forced vital capacity (FVC) and forced expiratory volume in 1 s (FEV_1). These improve following the administration of bronchodilators.
- The residual lung volume and total lung capacity are increased due to air trapping.

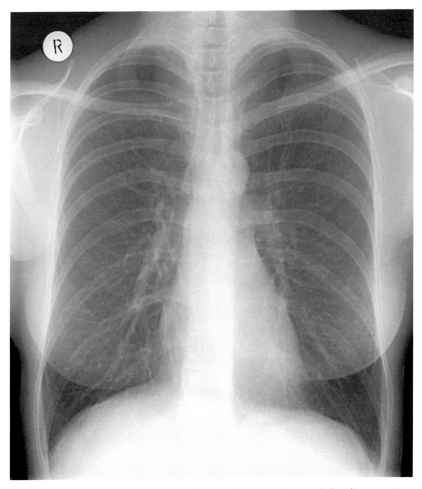

Asthma. The lungs are hyperinflated; there is bilateral diaphragmatic flattening; 7 anterior and 11 posterior ribs are visible; lungs are otherwise clear.

Radiological features

- Early in the disease the radiology may be entirely normal. Chronic asthma is associated with a number of distinct radiographic changes.
- **CXR** – lungs are hyperinflated with flattened hemidiaphragms of limited excursion. There is bronchial wall thickening (>1 mm). This is a more marked finding in children and in adults with infection. There is also hilar enlargement due to a combination of lymphadenopathy and pulmonary hypertension.
- **CT** may confirm thickened bronchi, but also areas of mosaic perfusion on 'lung windows'. These represent variable alternate areas of air trapping set against normally perfused and aerated lung.
- Always look for complications of asthma:
  - Pneumothorax or rarely pneumomediastinum.
  - Consolidation secondary to pulmonary infection.
  - Mucus plugging and subsequent lobar or segmental lung collapse.
  - In 2% allergic bronchopulmonary aspergillosis (ABPA) – dilated central bronchiectasis, with mucus plugging, associated with eosinophilia.

Differential diagnosis

- The radiological features are similar to those of cystic fibrosis.
- However the clinical mimics of asthma are important to differentiate. They can often be diagnosed with imaging and should be considered, particularly in atypical cases.
- Inhaled foreign body (particularly in children). Look for compatible history and asymmetric air trapping. CT imaging or bronchoscopy should be considered.
- Left heart failure. Look carefully for early interstitial pulmonary oedema.
- Tracheobronchial stenosis – tracheal narrowing will be visible on the CXR.
- Hypersensitivity pneumonitis – look for ground glass change and centrilobular nodules on CT.
- Post infectious bronchiolitis – air trapping on HRCT.

Management

- ABC.
- Bronchodilators – inhaled and nebulised (e.g. salbutamol).
- Inhaled steroids ± oral/IV steroids.
- Antibiotics.
- Physiotherapy.
- Early consideration for ventilatory support.
- Maintenance inhalers and good technique to prevent attacks.

Bochdalek hernia

Characteristics

- Congenital anomaly with defective fusion of the posterolateral pleuro-peritoneal layers.
- 85–90% on the left, 10–15% on the right. Usually unilateral lying posteriorly within the chest.
- Hernia may contain fat or intra-abdominal organs.
- In neonates the hernia may be large and present in utero. This is associated with high mortality secondary to pulmonary hypoplasia (60%).
- Small hernias are often asymptomatic containing a small amount of fat only. They have a reported incidence up to 6% in adults.

Clinical features

- Large hernias are diagnosed antenatally with US.
- Neonates may present with respiratory distress early in life. Early corrective surgery is recommended.
- Smaller hernias are usually asymptomatic with incidental diagnosis made on a routine CXR.
- Occasionally solid organs can be trapped within the chest compromising the vascular supply. Patients report localised pains and associated organ-related symptoms, e.g. change in bowel habit.

Radiological features

- **CXR** – a well-defined, dome-shaped soft tissue opacity is seen midway between the spine and the lateral chest wall. This may 'come and go'. There may be loops of bowel or gas-filled stomach within the area. The ipsilateral lung may be smaller with crowding of the bronchovascular markings and occasionally mediastinal shift. An NG tube may lie curled in the chest.
- **CT** – small hernia are difficult to demonstrate even on CT. Careful inspection for a fatty or soft tissue mass breaching the normal smooth contour of the posterior diaphragm.

Differential diagnosis

- In neonates, both congenital cystic adenomatoid malformation (CCAM) and pulmonary sequestration may have similar features. Cross-sectional imaging with CT ± MRI utilising 2D reformats is often very helpful.
- In adults, the plain film findings mimic pulmonary neoplasms, bronchogenic cysts and infections (± cavitation).

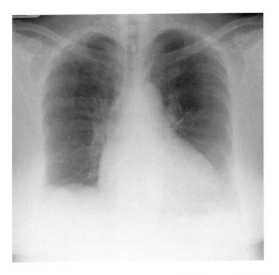

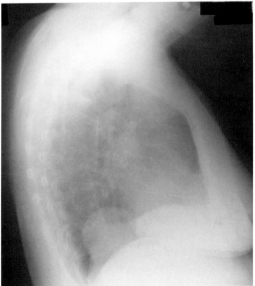

Bochdalek hernia. An apparent mass is present at the right lung base on the frontal radiograph. This is seen herniating through the posterior aspect of the right hemi-diaphragm on the lateral view; 10–15% of Bochdalek hernias occur on the right.

Management

- Large hernias in neonates require early surgical repair. They may also require respiratory support.
- In adults no active management is required in asymptomatic individuals.

Bronchiectasis

Characteristics

- Localised irreversible dilatation of bronchi often with thickening of the bronchial wall.
- **Congenital** – structural (bronchial atresia); abnormal mucociliary transport (Kartagener's); abnormal secretions (cystic fibrosis) or secondary to impaired immune system.
- **Acquired**
  - Post childhood infections.
  - Distal to bronchial obstruction (mucus plug, foreign body, neoplasm).
  - 'Traction bronchiectasis' secondary to pulmonary fibrosis.
- Types of bronchiectasis
  - Cylindrical or tubular (least severe type).
  - Varicose.
  - Saccular or cystic (most severe type).

Clinical features

- Most common presentation is in children.
- Increasing breathlessness.
- Chronic cough with excess sputum secretion.
- Haemoptysis.
- Recurrent chest infections with acute clinical exacerbations.

Radiological features

- Posterobasal segments of lower lobes most commonly affected.
- Bilateral in 50%.
- **CXR** – dilated, thick-walled bronchi giving cystic and tram-lining appearance particularly in the lower lobes. There may be volume loss and overt 'honeycombing'.
- There may be associated areas of infective consolidation and pleuro-parenchymal distortion.
- **HRCT** – lack of bronchial wall tapering is the most consistent feature. 'Signet ring' sign demonstrating a dilated bronchus adjacent to a smaller normal-calibre artery. The dilated bronchus extends out towards the pleura (<1 cm). Mucus plugging present.

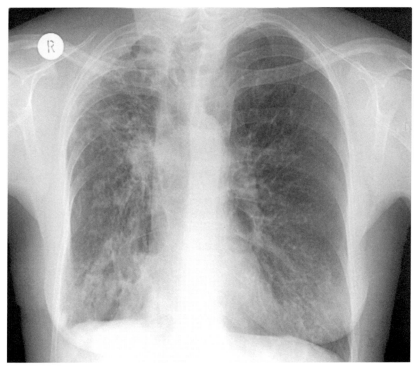

Bronchiectasis. There is widespread bronchial wall abnormality in both lungs, but particularly in the right lung. In the right lower zone, there is marked bronchial wall thickening (remember that the normal bronchial wall should be 'pencil line' thin) with 'tram lines' visible.

Differential diagnosis

- Bronchiectasis may be difficult to appreciate on plain films and even sometimes on CT.
- The main differential on plain films and CT lies with the honey-combing seen in advanced pulmonary fibrosis.
- On CT, bullous emphysema can mimic cystic bronchiectasis. However, expiratory films confirm air trapping in emphysema and a degree of airway collapse in bronchiectasis.

Management

- Regular postural physiotherapy with mucus drainage.
- Early use of antibiotics, sometimes with long-term prophylactic regimes.
- Bronchodilators may help in acute infective attacks associated with bronchospasm.

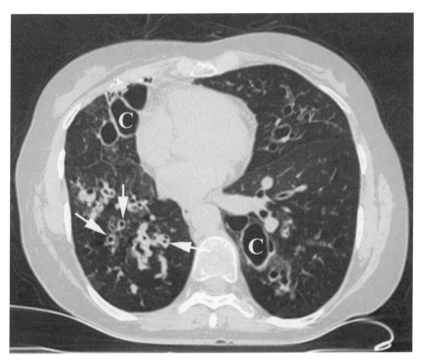

Bronchiectasis (HRCT). Widespread cystic dilatation of the bronchi (**C**), predominantly in the middle and left lower lobes. Note the marked bronchial wall thickening and several 'signet rings' (arrows) in the right lower lobe.

Bronchocele

Characteristics

- Mucoid impaction from accumulated inspissated secretions within the bronchial lumen. Usually associated with bronchial dilatation.
- Associated with bronchial obstruction – neoplasm, adenoma and atresia.
- Associated without bronchial obstruction – asthma, cystic fibrosis and infection.

Clinical features

- Variable symptoms including shortness of breath, cough, purulent sputum and haemoptysis. Some patients may be asymptomatic (e.g. bronchial atresia).
- There may be history of chronic illness.

Radiological features

- **CXR** – the lesion may be solitary or multiple, often measuring in excess of 1 cm in diameter with branching 'fingers' extending towards the periphery, the so-called gloved finger shadow. There may be air trapping and lucency distal to the bronchocele. Sometimes the obstructing lesion produces lung collapse, making it impossible to identify the bronchocele on CXRs.
- **CT** – confirms the plain film changes with dilated mucus-filled bronchi ± distal air trapping. The CT is very good for identifying obstructing neoplastic masses and demonstrating bronchoceles in a region of lung collapse.

Differential diagnosis

- The different potential causes of bronchoceles. A good clinical history coupled with cross-sectional imaging is usually diagnostic.

Management

- Removal of the obstructing lesion may be necessary. Bronchoscopy is a useful way of removing large mucus plugs and obtaining a tissue diagnosis from neoplastic masses.
- Non-obstructing lesions require physiotherapy and antibiotic administration.

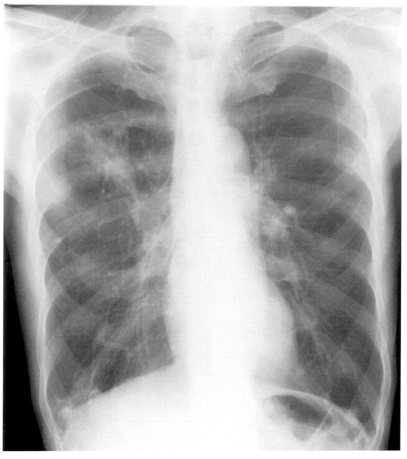

Bronchocele. Right upper lobe bronchocele.

Calcified granulomata

Characteristics

- Solitary or multiple calcified nodules within the lung. They are often small, widespread and punctate. Solitary granulomata, particularly post TB infection, can be large up to several centimetres in diameter.
- They represent a chronic healed immune reaction, within the lung, to the initial stimulus.
- Post infective causes – TB, post varicella pneumonia.
- Non-infectious causes – inhalation of organic and inorganic chemicals.

Clinical features

- Patients often asymptomatic.
- Previous history of infection or exposure to inhalational chemical.
- Can develop a non-productive cough and shortness of breath.
- Small risk of a pneumothorax.

Radiological features

- **CXR** – dense calcified sharply marginated pulmonary nodules. They can be solitary, multiple, localised or widespread. Distribution may correlate with the underlying cause, e.g. previous TB in the upper lobes.
- There is no growth in size of the calcified nodules over time.

Differential diagnosis

- Calcified lung metastases (e.g. breast, thyroid, osteosarcoma, ovarian, testicular and mucinous tumours). They can be multiple or solitary. They are often larger in size with an antecedent history supporting the primary neoplasm. Importantly they enlarge over time.
- ALWAYS COMPARE WITH OLD FILMS.
- If concerned repeat the CXR at an interval period in time.

Management

- No active management required.
- No surveillance necessary.

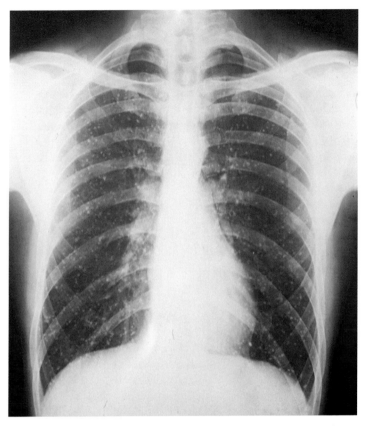

Calcified granulomata. Multiple calcified nodules scattered throughout both lungs.

Carcinoma

Characteristics

- Primary lung cancer represents the leading cause of cancer deaths in both males and females, and is the commonest cancer in males.
- Strong association with smoking, exposure to industrial chemicals (e.g. asbestos).
- Age of onset usually > 40, but beware aggressive forms in a younger age group.
- Three main subtypes
  - Small cell (most aggressive) (SCLC).
  - Non-small cell (squamous, large cell and adenocarcinoma) (NSCLC).
  - Bronchoalveolar cell carcinoma (BAC).
- Clinical management depends on disease extent (staging) and importantly tumour type.

Clinical features

- May be asymptomatic – identified on routine CXR.
- Any of the following symptoms, cough, SOB, wheeze and/or haemoptysis, raises the possibility of tumour presence.
- Chest pain, dysphagia or a hoarse voice from local extension of the tumour.
- Systemic upset – anorexia, cachexia, clubbing.
- Associated with metastatic spread – headaches, bone pain.
- Associated paraneoplastic syndromes with hormone release (Cushing's, acromegaly, gynaecomastia).

Radiological features

- **CXR** – solitary peripheral mass. Central in 40%. The mass can be smooth or irregular in outline and can cavitate. Satellite nodules may be present. There may be hilar, paratracheal and/or mediastinal lymphadenopathy. Direct spread may result in rib destruction and extrathoracic extension. There may be distant rib metastases.
- Other **CXR** presentations include patchy consolidation that fails to respond to antibiotics (commonly BAC), pleural effusions, bronchoceles and lung collapse, which may be partial or complete (lobar/segmental).
- **CT** allows characterisation of the mass and full staging of the cancer
  - Size and location of the tumour.
  - Presence of lymphadenopathy.
  - Presence of metastases (bone, adrenals and liver).

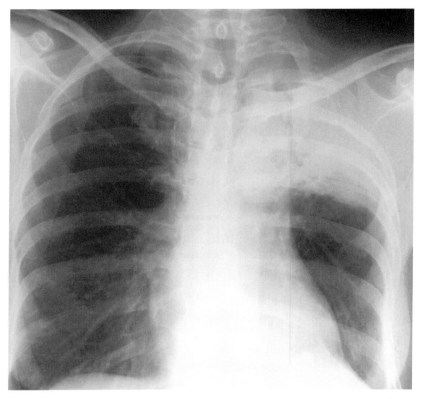

Carcinoma with rib destruction. Dense opacification of the left upper lobe with associated destruction of the left second and third anterior ribs.

• **PET/CT** – increased uptake of FDG tracer in primary cancer and metastases. Sensitive tool for staging tumours and discriminating ambiguous mass lesions.

Differential diagnosis (solitary pulmonary nodule)

• Neoplasms – lymphoma, carcinoid, hamartoma and solitary metastasis.
• Inflammatory
  • Infective – granuloma, pneumonia or abscess.
  • Non-infective – rheumatoid arthritis, sarcoid, Wegener's.
• Congenital – arteriovenous malformation, pulmonary sequestration.
• Miscellaneous – pulmonary infarct, rounded atelectasis.

Management

• Compare with old films – beware slow-growing squamous cell carcinomas.
• Tissue diagnosis is important – either with bronchoscopy or percutaneous biopsy (>90% sensitivity) of the primary tumour or metastatic deposit.
• Full tumour staging.
• Consideration for surgical resection (potentially curative) and/or chemoradiotherapy.
• Palliative treatment of symptoms (pain and hypercalcaemia).
• Screening has not shown any benefit in the early detection and treatment of lung cancer.

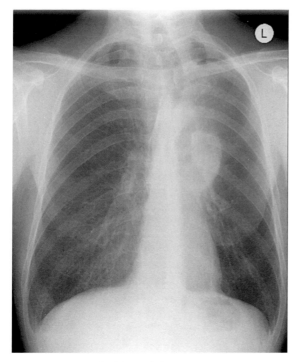

Left hilar carcinoma – CXR. Left hilar mass resulting in left upper lobe collapse.

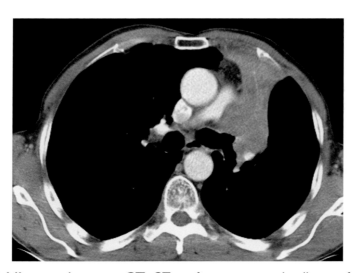

Left hilar carcinoma – CT. CT confirms segmental collapse of the left upper lobe, secondary to an obstructing carcinoma at the left hilum.

Cardiac aneurysm

Characteristics

- A true aneurysm is a circumscribed non-contractile outpouching of the left ventricle.
- Although there is a very rare congenital form, the majority occur as a complication of myocardial infarction. It rarely ruptures, but patients are at risk of arrhythmias and thromboembolic events that occur from clot formation within the aneurysm.
- A pseudoaneurysm, or false cardiac aneurysm, occurs acutely following trauma or a myocardial infarction, with a focal left ventricular rupture, localised haematoma and a high risk of delayed rupture and death.

Clinical features

- Most are asymptomatic and go without any problems.
- There is an association with arrhythmias, thromboembolic events and rarely cardiac failure.

Radiological features

- **CXR** – localised bulge in the left heart border. There is often a thin peripheral rim of calcification within the ventricular wall.
- **Echocardiography** – paradoxical movement of the left ventricular wall in systole is diagnostic. The aneurysm may contain thrombus.

Differential diagnosis

- Previous TB pericarditis, with a background of ischaemic heart disease, can have a very similar appearance on a frontal CXR. A lateral view may show absence of the localised posterior LV aneurysm. Echocardiography allows accurate characterisation of both pathologies.

Management

- No active treatment necessary.
- Occasionally anticoagulation for mural thrombus formation is needed.

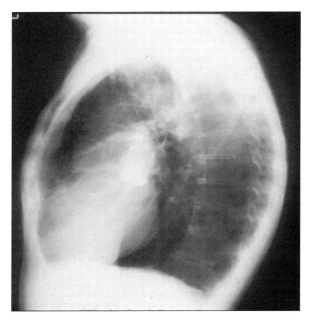

Fig. (cont.)

Coarctation of the aorta

Characteristics

- Congenital narrowing at the junction of the aortic arch and descending aorta, secondary to a fibrous ridge protruding into the aortic lumen.
- 80% male.
- 50% associated with other congenital anomalies:
  - Bicuspid aortic valve.
  - Turner's syndrome.
  - PDA, VSD.
  - Cerebral Berry aneurysms.
- Second most common cause of cardiac failure in neonates.
- May remain undetected well into adult life.

Clinical features

- Symptomatic presentation in neonates includes tachypnoea, cyanosis and generalised oedema. Patients require urgent corrective surgery. Most cases are now identified on neonatal screening.
- Delayed presentation in adults includes hypertension, headaches, claudication, cardiac failure and renal impairment.
- Patients may have cardiac systolic heart murmurs sometimes heard over the back and 'pistol shot' femoral pulses.

Radiological features

- Neonates – cardiomegaly and pulmonary plethora.
- Adults – **CXR**
  - Inferior rib notching (ribs 3–9), may be unilateral depending on where the right subclavian branches from the aorta. Only visible after 7 years of age.
  - Small aortic knuckle.
  - Figure-3 indentation on the left lateral wall of the aortic arch. The reverse-3 is present on barium studies.
  - Elevated left ventricular apex secondary to hypertrophy.
- **MRI** is very good at characterising the coarctation and associated cardiac anomalies.
- The extent of the stenosis is very difficult to assess on imaging.

Differential diagnosis

- Pseudo-coarctation – no pressure gradient across a narrowing in the aortic calibre – no obstruction.

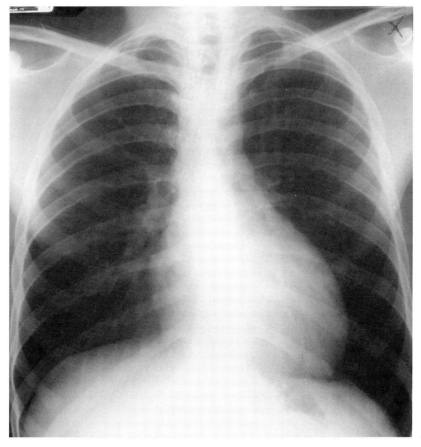

Coarctation of aorta. Note the rib notching and the 'figure of 3' arch of aorta

- Inflammatory conditions such as Takayasu's arteritis can have similar radiological features.
- Chronic SVC, IVC or subclavian artery obstruction may have similar radiological features.

Management

- Angioplasty and stenting.
- Surgical repair.
- Hypertension control.

Collapsed lung

Characteristics

- Lung collapse or atelectasis can affect the whole lung, a single lobe or a segmental component. The lobar collapses are important not to miss on imaging. They may be associated with an underlying malignancy.
- Causes are either obstructive or non-obstructive.
- Obstructive
  - Tumour which may lie outside or inside the bronchus or within the bronchial wall.
  - Foreign body.
  - Mucus plug.
  - Stricture – inflammatory, amyloidosis.
  - Bronchial rupture.
- Non-obstructive
  - Pleural effusions and pulmonary fibrosis.

Clinical features

- SOB, cough, haemoptysis, purulent sputum.
- Patients may be asymptomatic.
- Patients may have symptoms related to an underlying systemic condition including weight loss, cachexia, anorexia and night sweats.

Radiological features

- It is important to recognise the common lobar collapses on a frontal **CXR**.
- Significantly in adults upper lobe collapse is almost always associated with primary lung malignancy (>95%).
- **Left upper lobe** – veiled opacification throughout the left hemithorax with obscuration of the left heart border. Visible left margin of the aortic arch (Luftsichel sign). Horizontal orientation and splaying of the lower lobe bronchovascular markings. Almost all cases have a proximal tumour which may only be visible on **CT** scans.
- **Left lower lobe** – reduced lung volume. Small left hilum. Triangular density behind the heart with obscuration of the medial aspect of the left hemidiaphragm. Bronchial reorientation in a vertical direction.
- **Right upper lobe** – reduced lung volume. Elevated right hilum. Triangular density abutting right medial mediastinum. A mass lesion at the right hilum may be present (Golden – S sign).
- **Right middle lobe** – obscuration of the right heart border. A **lateral CXR** may be necessary to confirm the collapse.

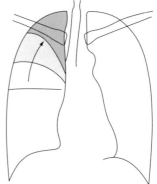

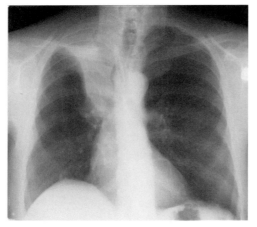

RUL collapse – PA.

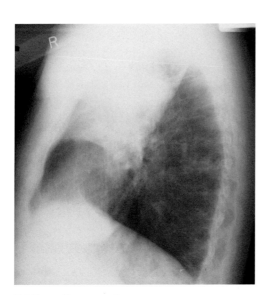

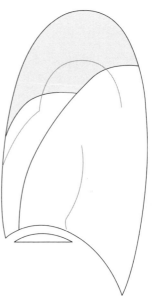

RUL collapse – Lat.

- **Right lower lobe** – Reduced lung volume. Triangular density medially at the right base obscuring the medial aspect of the right hemidiaphragm. Bronchial reorientation in a vertical direction.
- **Total lung collapse** – causes include misplaced endotracheal tube or large proximal tumour. Opacification of affected hemithorax with mediastinal shift to the collapsed lung.

Differential diagnosis

- Lobar consolidation may have similar appearances. Lateral chest films and the demonstration of lung volume loss in collapse are diagnostic.
- Hiatus hernias may mimic lower lobe collapse.
- Post pneumonectomy lungs may demonstrate volume loss and bronchial reorientation.

Management

- Bronchoscopy may be both diagnostic and in some cases therapeutic.
- CT scan to confirm underlying cause.
- In malignant collapse, radiotherapy and bronchial stenting can be of benefit.

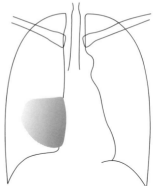

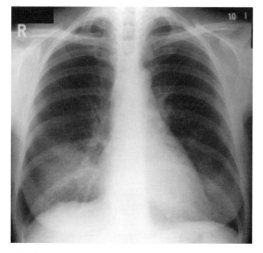

RML collapse – PA.

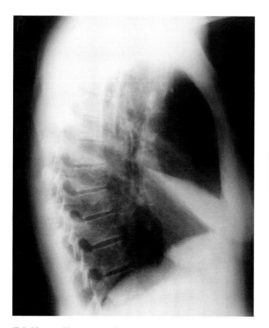

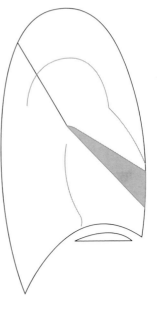

RML collapse – Lat.

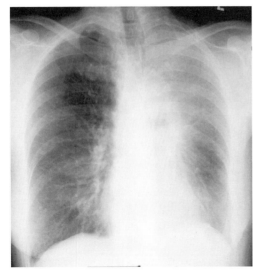
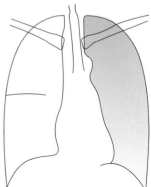

LUL collapse – **PA**.

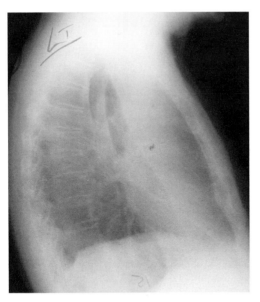
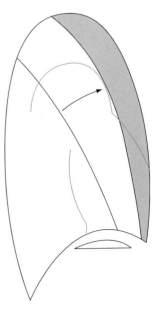

LUL collapse – **Lat**.

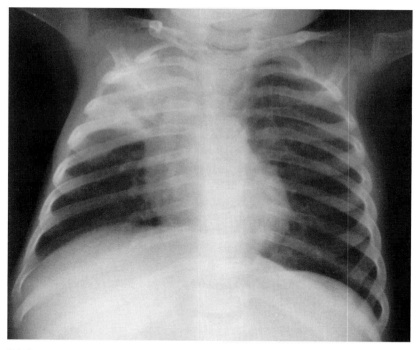

Right upper lobe consolidation. Dense opacification in the right upper zone containing air bronchograms.

Radiological features

- **May lag behind clinical onset and remain after resolution!**
- **CXR**
  - **Lobar pneumonia** – opacification of a lobe; usually *Streptococcus*. Air bronchograms may be present.
  - **Primary TB** – right paratracheal (40%) and right hilar adenopathy (60%) with consolidation in the mid or lower zones.
  - **Post primary TB** – ill-defined consolidation in the apical segments which may cavitate.
  - **Right middle and lower lobe pneumonia** – loss of the outline of the right heart border and the right hemidiaphragm silhouette respectively.
  - **Lingular segment pneumonia** – loss of the outline of the left heart border.
  - **Left lower lobe consolidation** – typically obliterates an arc of left hemidiaphragm. Look 'through the heart' for loss of diaphragmatic outline.
- FOLLOW–UP IMAGING IN ADULTS ESSENTIAL.
- FAILURE TO RESPOND TO ANTIBIOTICS MAY MEAN ANOTHER DIAGNOSIS SHOULD BE CONSIDERED.

Differential diagnosis

- Bronchoalveolar carcinoma.
- Lymphoma.
- Inflammatory conditions (Wegener's granulomatosis).
- Cryptogenic organising pneumonia.
- Cardiac failure.
- Sarcoid.

Management

- Most patients can be discharged with appropriate oral antibiotics.
- Give advice regarding deep breathing and coughing.
- A NSAID may be of benefit in patients with pleuritic pain to enable deep breathing and coughing.
- Treat the unwell patient with high flow oxygen (remember the patient with COPD is often dependent on their hypoxic drive to stimulate respiration), IV fluids, IV antibiotics ± analgesia.
- Follow-up imaging in adults.

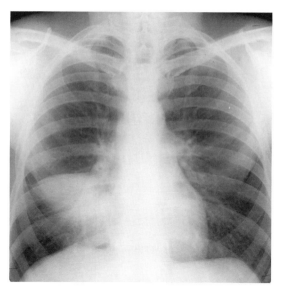

Right middle lobe consolidation – PA. Dense opacification in the right mid zone; this abuts the horizontal fissure and effaces the right heart border.

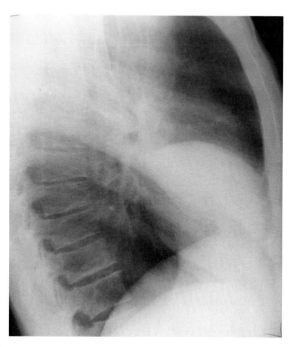

Right middle lobe consolidation – Lat. The density lies between the horizontal and oblique fissures – the position of the middle lobe.

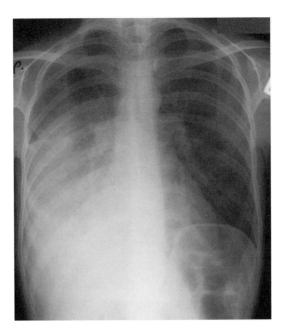

Right lower lobe consolidation – PA. Dense opacification in the right lower zone with effacement of the outline of the right hemi-diaphragm.

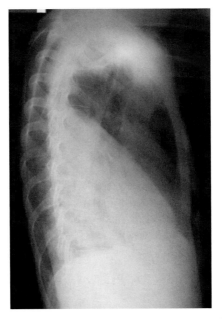

Right lower lobe consolidation – Lat. The density lies posterior to the oblique fissure – the position of the lower lobe.

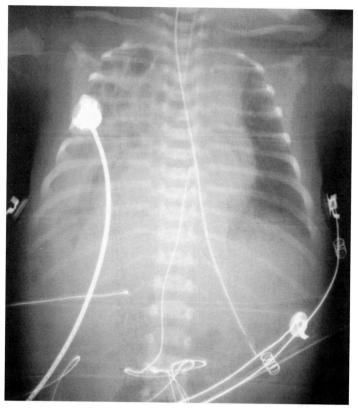

Congenital diaphragmatic hernia. This is a neonatal film. The right lung is opacified with multiple air-filled loops of bowel.

Embolic disease

Characteristics

- Pulmonary thromboembolism is a complication of deep vein thrombosis.
- If untreated there is a 30% mortality. If treated the mortality falls to <5%.
- Highest cause of maternal mortality in pregnancy.
- Associated with malignancy, immobility, thrombotic haematological disorders.
- D–Dimer blood test is very sensitive, but not very specific.
- Treatment is aimed at preventing further emboli.
- Patients with recurrent emboli may require long-term, sometimes lifelong, warfarin.
- Rarely emboli may represent fat emboli (following extensive lower limb/pelvic trauma) or tumour emboli. Fat embolus is rare and a distinct phenomenon. Patients present with acute SOB/collapse and dramatic CXR changes (extensive bilateral air space opacification similar to ARDS – adult respiratory distress syndrome).

Clinical features

- SOB.
- Cough, haemoptysis.
- Pleuritic chest pain.
- Deep leg vein thrombus.
- Hypoxia.
- Hypotension, tachycardia.
- Pulmonary arterial hypertension with right heart strain and failure.
- Collapse.
- Sudden death.

Radiological features

- **CXR** – may be normal.
- Other radiographic features of pulmonary embolic disease include:
  - Fleischner's sign – local widening of pulmonary artery due to distension from clot.
  - Hampton's hump – segmental pleurally based wedge-shaped opacity representing a pulmonary infarct.
  - Westermark's sign – peripheral wedge-shaped lucency due to focal lung oligaemia.
- **Ventilation/perfusion scan** – mismatched perfusion defects.

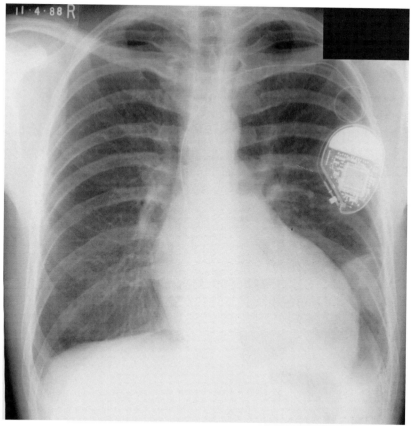

Pulmonary emboli. A peripheral wedge-shaped density is seen in the left lower zone; representing a pulmonary infarct. This appearance is known as a 'Hampton's hump'.

- **CT scan (CTPA)** – filling defects within the pulmonary arterial tree on contrast-enhanced imaging. There may also be mosaic perfusion with reduced vasculature in the lucent areas.
- **Pulmonary angiography** – filling defects.
- **Echocardiography** – dilated right atrium with right ventricular hypertrophy and pulmonary arterial hypertension.

Differential diagnosis

- The clinical presentation and CXR features are often non-specific and a number of conditions may mimic embolic disease (e.g. pneumothorax, infection, asthma and lung neoplasms).

Management

- ABC.
- Oxygen.
- Anticoagulation if PE is confirmed.
- Extensive thromboemboli with hypotension and tachycardia may require treatment with thrombolysis.

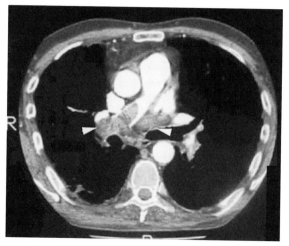

Pulmonary emboli – CTPA. Large filling defects (arrowheads), representing emboli, are seen in the main pulmonary arteries.

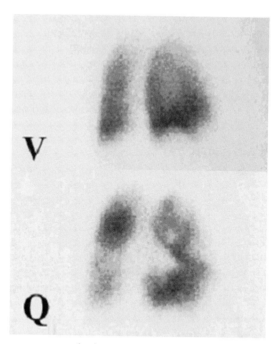

Pulmonary emboli – $\dot{V}/\dot{Q}$. This demonstrates '$\dot{V}/\dot{Q}$ mismatch' – an abnormality of perfusion ($\dot{Q}$) against a background of normal ventilation ($\dot{V}$).

Emphysematous bulla

Characteristics

- Abnormal permanent enlargement of distal air spaces with destruction of alveolar walls ± lung fibrosis. Overlaps with chronic bronchitis to form a disease spectrum known as chronic obstructive pulmonary disease.
- Due to an imbalance between lung proteases and anti-proteases.
- A bulla is an avascular low attenuation area that is larger than 1 cm and has a thin but perceptible wall.
- Associated with smoking but other chemicals and genetic disorders predispose to the condition (e.g. alpha–1 antitrypsin deficiency).
- Three types of emphysema
  - Panacinar, centrilobular and paraseptal.
- The different types of emphysema may coexist.

Clinical features

- May be asymptomatic, early in the disease.
- Exacerbations commonly precipitated by infection.
- Cough, wheeze and exertional dyspnoea.
- Tachypnoea, wheeze, lip pursing (a form of PEEP), use of accessory muscles (patients are referred to as pink puffers).
- Signs of hypercarbia include coarse tremor, bounding pulse, peripheral vasodilatation, drowsiness, confusion or an obtunded patient.

Radiological features

- **CXR** – focal area of well-defined lucency outlined with a thin wall. A fluid level may indicate infection within the bulla.
- Other **CXR** features include hyperexpanded lungs with associated flattening of both hemi-diaphragms, 'barrel-shaped chest', coarse irregular lung markings (thickened dilated bronchi – chronic bronchitis overlaps) and enlargement of the central pulmonary arteries in keeping with pulmonary arterial hypertension.
- REMEMBER to look for lung malignancy/nodules; a common association.
- **CT** quantifies the extent, type and location of emphysema. It may also identify occult malignancy.

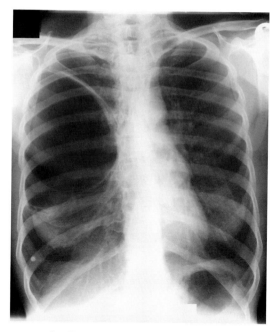

Emphysematous bulla. A large hypo-dense area, devoid of lung markings, is seen occupying most of the right lung. This compresses adjacent lung parenchyma.

Differential diagnosis

- Post-infective pneumatoceles.
- Loculated pneumothorax.
- Oligaemia secondary to pulmonary emboli or hilar vascular compression.

Management

- Emphysematous bullae form part of a spectrum of chronic obstructive pulmonary disease (see p. 62).
- Bullae in their own right usually need no active treatment. However, if severe disease, lung reduction surgery should be considered.

Extrinsic allergic alveolitis

Characteristics

- Also known as hypersensitivity pneumonitis.
- Represents an abnormal, exaggerated immune response to an inhaled organic allergen.
- Acute, subacute and chronic forms.
- Symptoms can develop after single or repeated exposures.
- Mixed type III and type IV immune reactions.
- Specific common antigens lead to specific conditions, e.g. farmer's lung (mouldy hay) and bird fancier's lung (droppings and feathers).

Clinical features

- Diagnosis is made from a combination of clinical history, radiological features, exposure to antigen and improvement following the withdrawal of the causative antigen.
- Occurs at any age, usually middle age depending on opportunity for antigen exposure.
- 90% positive precipitating serum antigens (however, this only reflects exposure to the antigen and not definite evidence for the association of EAA).
- History may be acute, 4 h after exposure – dry cough, fever, SOB, malaise. Symptoms can resolve immediately after withdrawal of the causative antigen.
- Subacute and chronic forms – months to years to develop. Main symptom is progressive, insidious breathlessness.

Radiological features

- Propensity for the middle lung zones, with sparing of the costophrenic angles and absolute apices.
- Radiology depends on the acute or chronic forms.
- **CXR**
  - Acute and subacute forms may be normal: patchy ground glass change and nodularity can be seen.
  - In the chronic form, fibrosis and parenchymal distortion are prominent features affecting the mid and upper zones.
- **HRCT**
  - Small round centrilobular nodules, with patchy ground glass attenuation and air trapping (mosaic perfusion).
  - Progression to the chronic form leads to interstitial thickening, honeycombing and traction bronchiectasis.

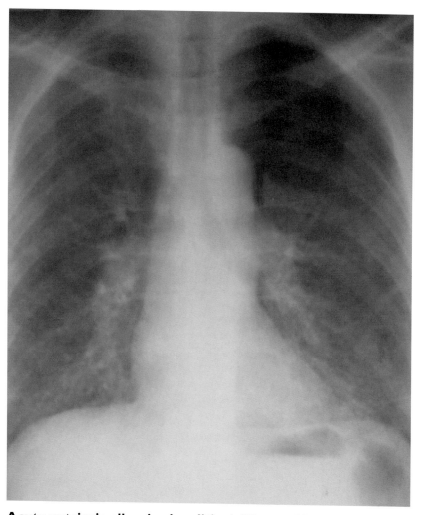

Acute extrinsic allergic alveolitis. A 37-year-old bird keeper, who had a 2-month history of cough, wheeze and mild SOB lasting for a few hours each day.

There are bilateral small ill-defined ground glass nodules throughout both lungs. The features are non-specific and may represent infective changes, but the history and X-ray features are typical of a hypersensitivity pneumonitis (or acute EAA).

Differential diagnosis

- Acute/subacute form
  - Infections, particularly TB and viral.
  - Obliterative bronchiolitis.
  - Chronic pulmonary embolic disease.
  - Early pulmonary metastatic disease.
- Chronic
  - Pulmonary fibrosis, e.g. UIP.
  - Chronic sarcoid.

Management

- Removal of causative inhalational antigen.
- Steroids may help some individuals.

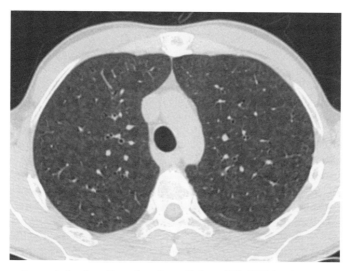

Subacute extrinsic allergic alveolitis – HRCT. Multiple small round centrilobular nodules throughout both lungs. Note the patchy air trapping (mosaic attenuation) within the left lung.

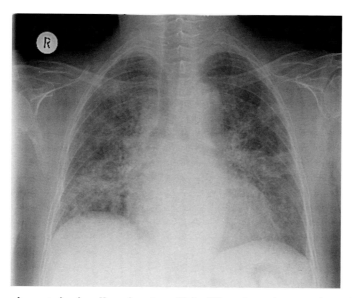

Chronic extrinsic allergic alveolitis. Fibrosis and parenchymal distortion are prominent within both mid zones and right lower zone.

Flail chest

Characteristics

- Occurs when there is loss of continuity of a segment of chest wall with the rest of the thoracic cage.
- Follows trauma, with two or more ribs fractured in two or more places.
- Results in disruption of normal chest wall movements, and paradoxical movement may be seen.
- Always consider underlying lung injury (pulmonary contusion).
- The combination of pain, decreased or paradoxical chest wall movements and underlying lung contusion are likely to contribute to the patient's hypoxia.
- High association with other accompanying traumatic injuries.

Clinical features

- Dyspnoea and hypoxia.
- Tachycardia.
- Cyanosis.
- Tachypnoea.
- Hypotension.
- Chest wall bruising ± palpable abnormal movement or rib crepitus.
- The degree of hypoxia often depends on the severity of the underlying pulmonary contusion.

Radiological features

- **CXR**
  - Multiple rib fractures.
  - Costochondral separation may not be evident.
  - Air space shadowing may be seen with pulmonary contusion (often absent on initial films).
  - There may be a pneumothorax, haemopneumothorax or lung collapse.

Differential diagnosis

- Simple rib fractures and pulmonary contusion with under ventilation secondary to chest wall pain.

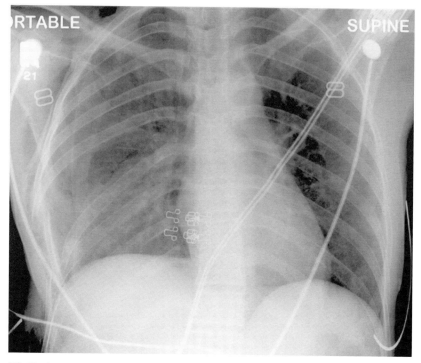

Flail chest – case 1. Multiple right-sided rib fractures. Note the double fracture of the right fifth rib.

Management

- Initial management includes securing the airway and maximising oxygenation.
- In the absence of systemic hypotension, judicious fluid replacement is required as the injured lung is susceptible to both under resuscitation and fluid overload.
- Definitive treatment includes oxygenation and adequate analgesia to optimise ventilation/lung re-expansion.
- A pleural drain or ventilatory support may be necessary.
- Treat associated injuries.

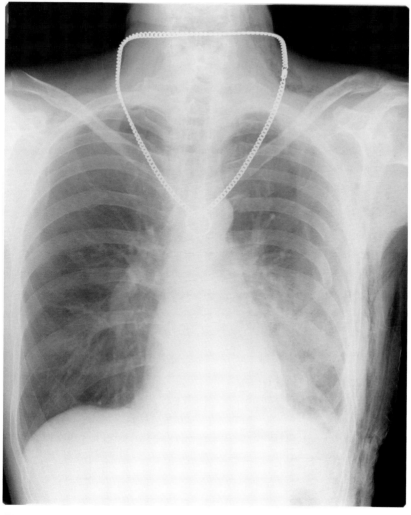

Flail chest – case 2. Double fractures of the left posterior fifth and sixth ribs.

Foregut duplication cyst

Characteristics

- This is a broad term used to encompass a number of congenital mediastinal cysts derived from the embryological foregut. They include bronchogenic, oesophageal duplication and neuroenteric cysts.
- Bronchogenic cysts are the most common and are thin-walled cysts lined by respiratory epithelium lying within the mediastinum.
- Foregut cysts are often picked up incidentally.
- Symptoms are due to compression of local structures or secondary to cyst haemorrhage or infection. Rarely, in children symptoms can be quite severe particularly in neonates.

Clinical features

- Most are asymptomatic.
- Can present with chest pain, dysphagia, wheeze and shortness of breath.
- In children they can be large and, if the cyst grows, complications from airway compression can be life threatening.

Radiological features

- **CXR** – spherical or oval mass with smooth outlines projected either side of the mediastinum. Most are unilocular. They are usually located in the middle mediastinum adjacent to the carina. They tend to push the carina forward and oesophagus posteriorly which is almost unique to foregut cysts.
- **CT** demonstrates a water density cyst (HU 0). Occasionally high protein content or infection can cause soft tissue attenuation within a cyst. This can cause diagnostic difficulty. Wall enhancement suggests infection.
- **MRI** is also a good way of demonstrating the location and contents of the cyst.

Differential diagnosis

- Pancreatic pseudocyst.
- Neurogenic tumour.
- Primary or secondary lung malignancy
- Lymphadenopathy, particularly necrotic tuberculous lymph nodes.

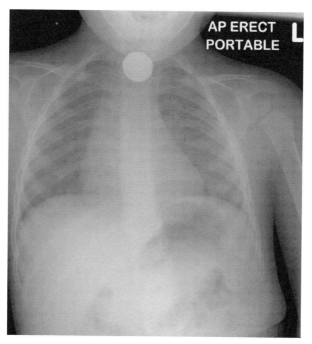

Swallowed foreign body.

Management

- Visualisation, both direct and indirect, is useful and may allow removal of a visible foreign body.
- Refer patients who are symptomatic, and for whom an obvious cause cannot be seen and removed.
- Endoscopy allows definitive management.
- Beware of patients swallowing potentially dangerous items such as button batteries (e.g. watch batteries) and sharp objects such as razor blades!
- In a child, a chest radiograph should be performed to demonstrate the site of the object. An abdominal X-ray is required if the object is not seen within the chest to both confirm passage into the abdomen, and for transit monitoring if the object does not appear in the stool after 1 to 2 days.

Goitre

Characteristics

- A goitre represents enlargement of the thyroid gland in the neck. It can be diffuse, multinodular or simply relate to an enlarged solitary nodule.
- Symptoms may be due to local mass effect, from thyroid hormonal imbalance or rarely due to the presence of a focal malignancy within the thyroid.
- The enlarged thyroid may extend from the neck inferiorly into the superior mediastinum and retrosternal region.
- Goitres are the most common mediastinal mass.
- More common in females and in middle-aged/older people.

Clinical features

- Most are asymptomatic, identified incidentally on a routine CXR.
- Symptoms may be due to local compression of the trachea or oesophagus. Occasionally recurrent laryngeal nerve palsies occur.
- Patients may be euthyroid, hyperthyroid or hypothyroid.
- Rarely a malignancy may coexist. Local pain and metastases can be a feature.

Radiological features

- **CXR** – superior soft tissue mass, which may extend into the neck or retrosternally. There may be tracheal deviation away from the mass or tracheal compression. The mass may have a smooth or lobulated appearance and contain foci of calcification.
- **CT** – the mass is usually of high attenuation, contains calcification and enhances avidly.

Differential diagnosis

- **4 Ts**
  - **T**hymus or **T**hymoma.
  - Germ cell tumour (e.g. **T**eratoma).
  - Lymphoma (e.g. **T**-cell lymphoma).
- If clinical doubt persists then biopsy and tissue sampling may be necessary.

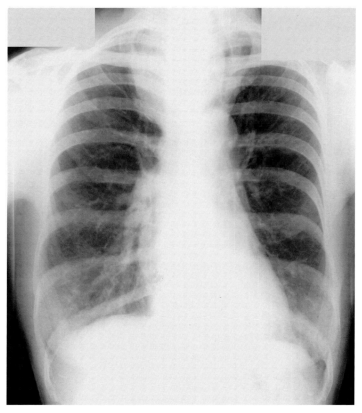

Goitre. Superior mediastinal mass extending into the neck, resulting in marked narrowing and displacement of the trachea to the left.

Management

- Most require no active treatment.
- If symptomatic patients should be considered for surgical resection (partial or complete thyroidectomy).
- Thyroid replacement hormone may be needed following surgery.

Haemothorax

Characteristics

- Accumulation of blood within the pleural space following blunt or penetrating trauma.
- Commonly associated with a pneumothorax and other extra-thoracic injuries.
- Haemorrhage usually occurs from the lung parenchyma, and is often self limiting, rather than from a specific vessel injury. Intercostal and internal mammary vessels are more commonly injured than the hilar or great vessels.

Clinical features

- Depends mainly on the amount of blood lost.
- Varying degrees of hypovolaemic shock.
- Breath sounds may be reduced or absent with dull percussion.

Radiological features

- Erect **CXR** is more sensitive than a supine film.
  - Blunting of the costophrenic angles – seen with approximately 250 ml of blood.
  - General increased opacification of the hemithorax is seen on a supine film.

Differential diagnosis

- Long-standing or acute pleural effusions (e.g. heart failure) may mimic a haemothorax. Review of old films and the clinical history is helpful. A pleural tap is diagnostic.

Management

- ABC with IV access prior to tube thoracostomy.
- Definitive management involves the placement of a large-bore tube thoracostomy. This allows both re-expansion of lung as well as estima-tion of initial and ongoing blood loss. Airway control and circulatory volume support are essential alongside definitive treatment. A patient with initial drainage of 1500 ml or greater than 200 ml/h is likely to require thoracotomy. Discuss with thoracic team and be guided by the patient's physiological status.

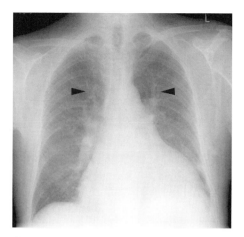

Stage 1 left heart failure. *Raised pulmonary venous pressure.* Note the bilateral upper lobe blood diversion (arrowheads).

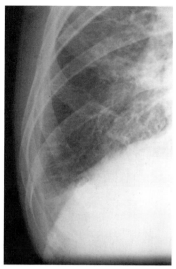

Stage 2 left heart failure. *Interstitial pulmonary oedema.* Prominent septal lines at the right costophrenic angle.

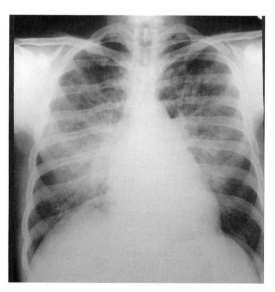

Stage 3 left heart failure. *Pulmonary oedema.* Bilateral perihilar ('bats wing') consolidation.

Hiatus hernia

Characteristics

- Two types:
  - **Sliding** (99%) – there is dehiscence of the diaphragmatic crura with herniation of the gastro-oesophageal junction (GOJ) above the diaphragm. The hernia can be very large and is often reducible in an upright position. Increased incidence with age.
  - **Rolling/paraoesophageal** (1%) – the GOJ lies at the level of the diaphragm. A part of the stomach herniates through the oesophageal opening in the diaphragm adjacent to the normal GOJ. The hernia rarely reduces.
- Both hernias increase with age. There is association with reflux oesophagitis. Both hernias predispose the stomach to volvulus. The rolling hernias are at high risk of incarceration.

Clinical features

- Often asymptomatic.
- Reflux indigestion. Food regurgitation. Coffee ground vomiting.
- Dysphagia.
- Epigastric or abdominal pain.

Radiological features

- **CXR**
  - May be normal.
  - Retrocardiac well demarcated soft tissue density. May be an air–fluid level.
  - Lateral film demonstrates an inferior, middle mediastinal soft tissue density mass, often with an air–fluid level.
- **Barium swallow**
  - The B–ring of the oesophagus lies above the diaphragm in sliding hiatus hernias. There may be narrowing at the B–ring with dilatation and often gastric mucosal folds lying above the diaphragm. There may be tertiary contractions and irregular mucosa due to reflux oesophagitis in the distal oesophagus.
  - A part of the stomach lies adjacent to the GOJ above the diaphragm in rolling hernias.
  - Both hernias predispose the stomach to volvulus.

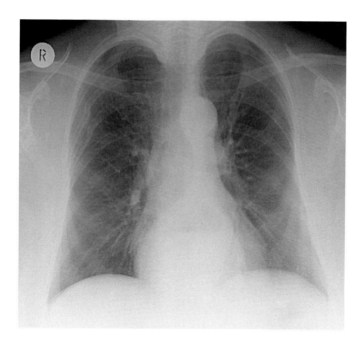

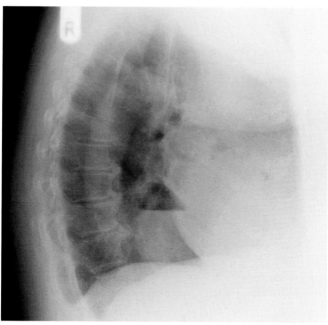

Hiatus hernia. There is a mass projected behind the heart in one of the 'hidden areas'. On the lateral view, an air-fluid level is seen confirming a hiatus hernia.

Differential diagnosis

- The differential diagnosis of a retrocardiac density on CXR includes posterior/middle mediastinal lesions:
  - Neurogenic tumour
  - Primary lung tumour
  - Thoracic aneurysm
  - GOJ cancer
  - Lymphadenopathy.

Management

- Often no treatment required.
- Long-term acid suppression with proton pump inhibitors.
- Surgical reduction of the hernia – Nissen fundoplication.

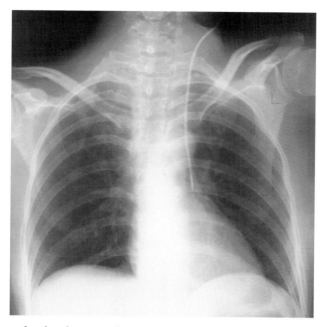

Incorrectly sited central venous line. This left internal jugular central venous line is incorrectly placed. The tip is directed directly into the mediastinum.

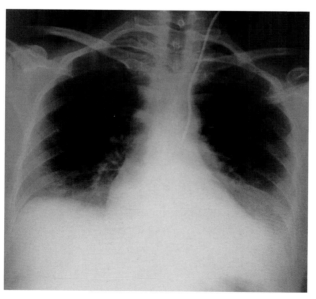

This error was not identified. When IV fluids were started this accumulated in the left pleural space.

Kartagener syndrome

Characteristics

- Rare syndrome associated with cilia dysmotility.
- Affects respiratory, auditory and sperm cilia.
- Triad of features
  - Situs inversus (50%).
  - Nasal polyposis and chronic sinusitis.
  - Bronchiectasis.
- Associated with deafness, infertility and other congenital anomalies (e.g. cardiac).
- Familial predisposition.

Clinical features

- Diagnosis in childhood. May be antenatal diagnosis.
- Dyspnoea, cough and sputum.
- Recurrent chest infections.

Radiological features

- **CXR** – dextrocardia ± situs inversus. Bibasal bronchiectasis. May be mucus plugging and lobar collapse or associated infective consolidation.
- **Facial X-ray** or **CT** – demonstrates extensive sinus soft tissue in keeping with polyps and mucus.

Differential diagnosis

- Cystic fibrosis and asthma may have similar appearances particularly as 50% of Kartagener's cases have no dextrocardia.

Management

- Chest physiotherapy.
- Long-term and/or recurrent antibiotic therapy.
- Consideration for heart-lung transplant.

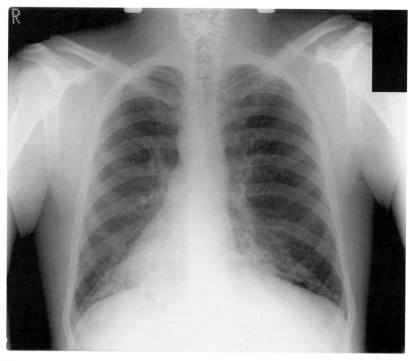

Kartagener syndrome. Dextrocardia and left lower lobe bronchiectasis.

Lymphangioleiomyomatosis

Characteristics

- This is a rare disease of unknown cause characterised by the presence of abnormal smooth muscle proliferation of the pulmonary interstitium, particularly in the bronchioles, pulmonary vessels and lymphatics.
- Exclusively affects women of a child-bearing age.
- Associated with chylous ascites, fatty liver and renal angiomyolipomas.

Clinical features

- Progressive exertional dyspnoea.
- Haemoptysis.
- Restrictive lung function and hypoxia.
- Increase in symptoms during pregnancy and on the oral contraceptive pill.

Radiological features

- **CXR** – coarse reticular interstitial pattern with cyst formation on the background of large volume lungs. There is a common association with chylous pleural effusions (70%), pneumothoraces (40%) and mediastinal lymphadenopathy.
- **HRCT** – numerous random thin-walled cysts of varying size and relatively regular shape. Bronchovascular bundles at edge of cyst. Lymphadenopathy, pleural effusions and pneumothoraces. Dilated thoracic duct.
- Long-standing cases may develop pulmonary arterial hypertension with enlargement of the central pulmonary arteries.

Differential diagnosis

- Langerhan's cell histiocytosis – male smokers, with upper zone predisposition and more cyst irregularity.
- Tuberous sclerosis – rare. Other characteristic abnormalities present.
- Emphysema – smokers. No wall to the emphysematous bullae.
- Neurofibromatosis – rare with musculoskeletal and neurogenic abnormalities.
- Lung fibrosis (e.g. UIP). Basal fibrosis and honeycombing.

Management

- Lung biopsy may be required to confirm the diagnosis.
- No specific treatment.
- 10-year survival is 75%.
- Progression to pulmonary insufficiency and arterial hypertension.

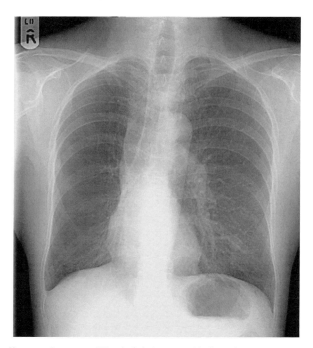

Macleod's syndrome. The left hilum and left pulmonary vascular tree appear normal. The right hilum is very small and the entire right hemithorax has a paucity of lung markings. Additional volume loss within the right lung. The right lung appears otherwise normal (i.e. it is not hypoplastic).

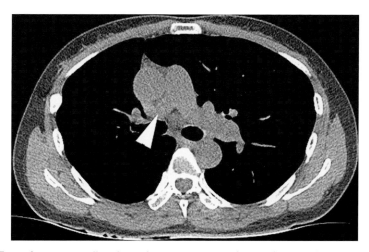

CT confirms a small right pulmonary artery (arrow) and additional volume loss within the right hemithorax.

Mastectomy

Characteristics

- Removal of the breast tissue in the treatment of breast cancer.
- Common form of treatment.
- It may be partial, or total, with additional removal of soft tissues from the chest wall and/or axilla.
- Reconstructive surgery or breast augmentation surgery with prostheses may be present.
- Patients receiving mastectomies often get adjuvant radiotherapy to the ipsilateral chest wall.

Clinical features

- Post mastectomy, the majority of patients are asymptomatic.
- Some patients may complain of chest wall discomfort.
- Clinicians should be alerted to the onset of new chest wall pain or chest symptoms (SOB, cough) as this may herald recurrent disease.

Radiological features

- **CXR**
  - Total mastectomy: there is increased transradiancy throughout the ipsilateral hemithorax. The axillary soft tissues may be reduced in thickness.
  - Partial mastectomy: may show breast shadow distortion or asymmetry of the breast shadows only.
  - Always look for changes consistent with radiotherapy in the bones (radionecrosis) which may mimic bone metastases.
  - There may be associated lung, pleural or bone metastases.

Differential diagnosis

- Poland's syndrome – congenital absence of pectoralis major.

Management

- No treatment required.

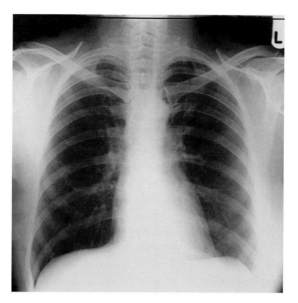

Right mastectomy.

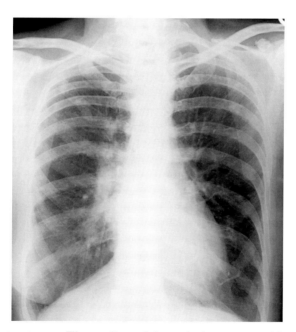

Left mastectomy. The outline of the right breast is visible whist the left is absent. In addition, the left hemithorax is hyper-transradiant as compared to the right.

Mesothelioma

Characteristics

- Benign and malignant forms.
- Most common malignant tumour of the pleura.
- Multiple tumour masses involving predominately the parietal pleura encasing the lung with a thick sheet-like tumour.
- Strong association with asbestos exposure. Also linked with chronic inflammation and irradiation.
- Can spread to the peritoneal pleura.
- Spread can be haematogenous or via the lymphatic route to lymph nodes, lung and liver.
- Presentation >50 years. M > F.

Clinical features

- Chest pain.
- Dyspnoea.
- Fever and sweats.
- Weakness and malaise.
- Cough.
- Weight loss.

Radiological features

- **CXR** – extensive lobulated pleural masses often extending over the mediastinal pleural surface. Volume loss in the lung. Associated pleural effusion. Pleural calcifications (25%). Extension into the interlobular fissures and rib destruction in 20%.
- **CT** – enhancing lobulated pleural thickening (>1 cm) encasing the lung. Extends over mediastinal surface. Associated lung nodules. Rib destruction and extrathoracic extension. Ascites is demonstrated in 30%.

Differential diagnosis

- Post infective pleural fibrosis.
- Post empyema.
- Pleural metastatic disease.

Management

- Confirm diagnosis with biopsy. Give radiation to biopsy site as tumour seeding occurs in 30%.

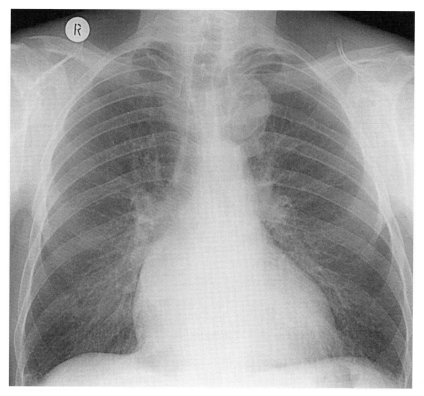

Neurofibromatosis. Large left superior mediastinal mass which can be placed within the posterior mediastinum:
- the left brachiocephalic vein is visible within the anterior mediastinum
- the left wall of the trachea is visible in the middle mediastinum.

- **MRI** – confirms the paravertebral soft tissue mass and demonstrates the intraspinal component giving rise to a 'dumb-bell tumour'. Further lesions both intra- and extra-spinally may also be demonstrated.
- Increase in size of lesions may represent malignant transformation.

Differential diagnosis

- Isolated neurogenic tumours (e.g. neuroblastoma or ganglioneuroma).
- Lateral meningocoele.
- Primary lung tumour.
- Bronchogenic cyst.
- Thoracic aortic aneurysm.
- Paraspinal abscess.
- Paraspinal extramedullary haematopoiesis.

Management

- May not require any treatment.
- Consider surgical excision of tumours if symptomatic.
- Follow-up screening of neurogenic tumours. There is a risk of malignant transformation, particularly if the tumour enlarges rapidly.

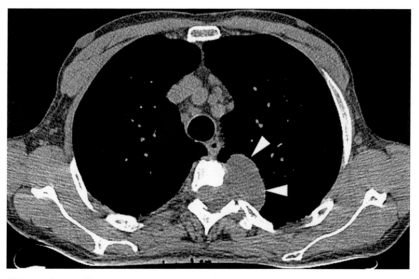

CT confirms the mass originates within the posterior mediastinum (arrows) and is continuous with the adjacent intervertebral foramen.

Pancoast tumour

Characteristics

- This is a primary lung tumour located in the lung apex.
- The majority are squamous cell carcinomas.
- They represent 3% of all primary lung tumours.
- Strong association with cigarette smoking.
- Usual age at presentation >40 years.
- The tumour spreads locally and patients often present with a specific set of signs and symptoms.

Clinical features

- May be asymptomatic.
- Chest and/or shoulder pain. Some patients are referred for a shoulder X-ray.
- Cough, sputum, haemoptysis.
- Weight loss and malaise.
- SVC obstruction.
- Hoarse voice.
- **Horner's syndrome** (enophthalmos, miosis, ptosis and anhidrosis) due to direct involvement of the sympathetic plexus.
- Wasting of the muscles in the hand and arm due to brachial plexus invasion.

Radiological features

- **CXR** – unilateral apical pleural thickening/mass. The mass lesion may cavitate. Hilar enlargement secondary to lymphadenopathy. May be rib destruction and extrathoracic soft tissue mass lesion.
- **CT** – confirms the apical mass lesion. Good for staging the tumour with assessment for mediastinal and metastatic disease.
- **MRI** – excellent for demonstrating local tissue invasion, particularly on T_1 sequences as extrathoracic spread and brachial plexus involvement are readily identified. Accurate assessment is needed prior to consideration for surgical excision.
- **PET/CT** – increased uptake of FDG tracer in primary cancer and metastases. Sensitive tool for staging tumours and discriminating ambiguous mass lesions.

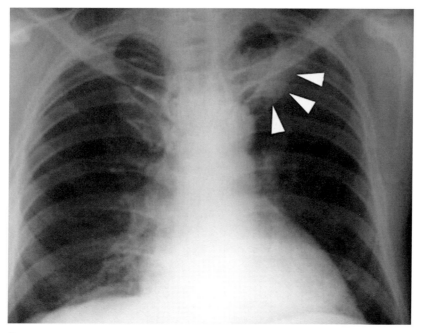

Pancoast tumour. Ill-defined tumour within the left apex
(arrowheads).

Differential diagnosis

- TB infection – this can represent active disease or simply be post infective pleuroparenchymal thickening.
- Fungal infection.
- Wegener's granulomatosis.

Management

- Sputum cytology.
- Transbronchial or transthoracic biopsy.
- Accurate staging.
- Radiotherapy.
- Surgical resection.

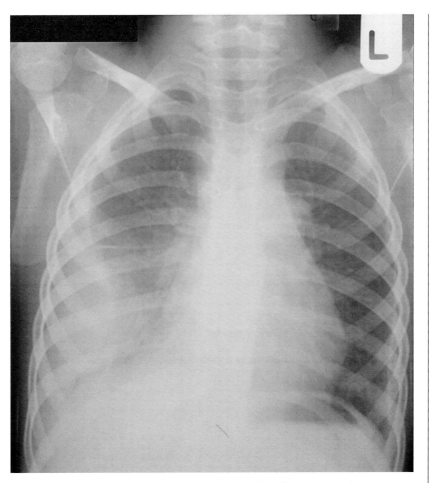

Lamellar pleural effusion. A meniscus of fluid is seen tracking up the right lateral chest wall beneath the loose connective tissue of the visceral pleura, typical of a lamellar effusion.

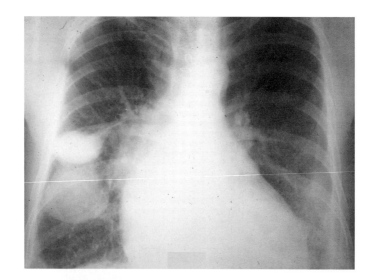

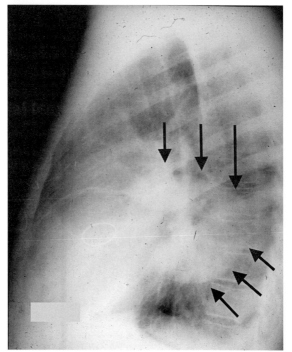

Encysted pleural effusions. Two well-marginated 'masses' within the right mid and lower zones. These are confirmed as encysted effusions within the horizontal and oblique fissures respectively, on the lateral view (arrows).

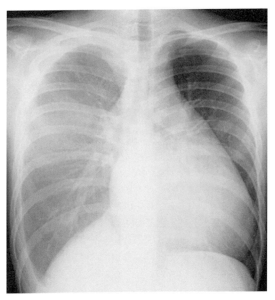

Right pleural effusion – supine film. The pleural fluid usually manifests as an increase in density within the affected hemithorax.

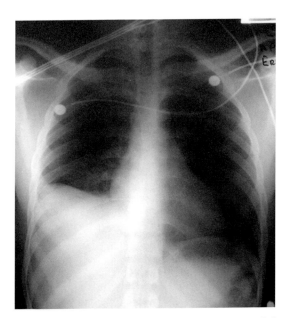

Subpulmonic pleural effusion. Apparent elevation of the right hemi-diaphragm, with the dome of the hemi-diaphragm shifted laterally and an acutely angled right costophrenic angle.

Pleural mass

Characteristics

- There are a number of conditions affecting the pleura which give rise to soft tissue pleural masses or the appearance of a pleural mass.
- **Benign** – pleural fibroma, pleural thickening or rounded atelectasis.
- **Malignant** – mesothelioma, metastases.
- The majority of pleural metastases are from lung or breast lesions, but other tumours including lymphoma, ovarian adenocarcinoma and plasmacytoma can either metastasise to or lie adjacent to the pleura giving the appearance of a pleural mass on imaging.
- A loculated empyema may resemble a pleural mass on routine imaging.
- Lastly, primary or secondary lung tumours can abut the pleura giving the appearance of a pleural mass.

Clinical features

- Benign – at least 50% are asymptomatic. Others present with cough, dyspnoea or chest pain.
  - Clubbing and hypertrophic pulmonary osteoarthropathy are not uncommon.
  - Rarely, symptomatic episodic hypoglycaemia is a recognised feature of pleural fibromas.
- Malignant lesions are usually more symptomatic.
  - Both SOB and chest wall pains are predominant features.
  - Weight loss and malaise accompany malignant disease.

Radiological features

- **CXR** – peripherally based soft tissue mass. Sharp medial margin with indistinct lateral margins. They may be multiple or solitary. Extra-thoracic soft tissue extension, rib destruction or lymphadenopathy suggests malignant disease.
- Pleural fibromas can be very large, up to 20 cm in diameter. They are pedunculated and can change position with posture.
- **CT** or **MRI** – confirms the pleurally based mass and characterises the presence of haemorrhage, calcification, multiplicity and local invasion.

Differential diagnosis

- The differential lies between discriminating true from apparent pleural masses and determining benign from malignant disease.

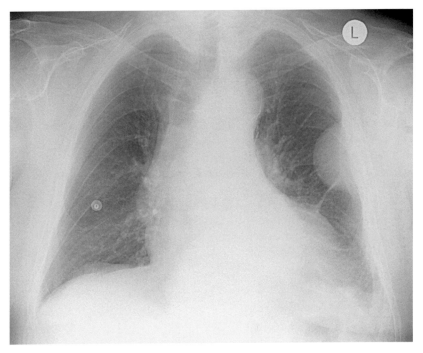

Pleural fibroma. Mass in the periphery of the left mid zone. This has a sharply defined medial border and an ill-defined lateral border, indicating that it is likely to be pleural in origin.

Management

- Management depends on the underlying cause.
- Investigation should be used to fully characterise the mass.
- In many cases no active treatment is required, particularly if benign and asymptomatic.
- Surgical excision for large masses.
- Radiotherapy can be used for malignant lesions.

Pneumoconiosis

Characteristics

- These represent a spectrum of lung conditions caused by inhalation of inorganic dust particles. The particles overwhelm the lung's defence mechanism and induce a chronic granulomatous reaction.
- The exposure to the particles occurs over many years.
- The resulting lung changes are progressive and irreversible.
- There are two main subtypes of pneumoconiosis:
  - Minimal symptoms as the particles are not fibrogenic, e.g. stannosis (tin), baritosis (barium) and siderosis (iron).
  - Symptomatic due to fibrogenic particles, e.g. silicosis (silica), asbestosis (asbestos) and coal workers' pneumoconiosis.
- All the conditions have very similar characteristic clinical and radiological features.

Clinical features

- May be asymptomatic.
- Non-productive cough.
- Dyspnoea – this is progressive.
- Weight loss, malaise.
- Hypoxia.
- Restrictive lung function.

Radiological features

- **CXR** – multiple bilateral 3- to 10-mm nodules present in the upper and mid zones. Some of the nodules coalesce. Different particles produce different density nodules, e.g. stannosis can be very dense. There may be hilar lymphadenopathy some of which show egg shell calcification. There may be fibrotic change and parenchymal distortion.
- **HRCT** – demonstrates small nodular opacities, interlobular septal thickening, fibrous parenchymal bands and a ground glass pattern.

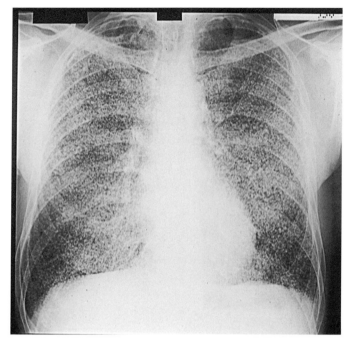

Pneumoconiosis – stannosis. Multiple small dense bilateral pulmonary nodules.

Differential diagnosis

- Sarcoidosis.
- TB.
- Post viral infections.
- Miliary metastases.
- Pulmonary alveolar microlithiasis.

Management

- No effective active treatment.

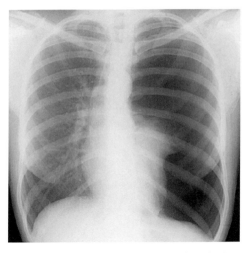

Tension pneumothorax – case 1. Large left-sided pneumothorax with early mediastinal shift to the right. This medical emergency is a clinical diagnosis and not a radiological one.

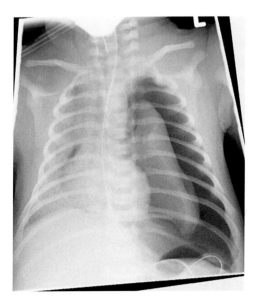

Tension pneumothorax – case 2. This is not an infrequent complication of ventilation.
The barotrauma associated with ventilation results in accumulation of air within the pleural space with limited egress of air. As a result, there is mediastinal shift away from the side of the pneumothorax. Associated deep sulcus sign. This is a medical emergency.

Poland's syndrome

Characteristics

- Congenital absence of the pectoralis major muscle.
- May be associated with ipsilateral absence of the pectoralis minor muscle, rib and arm anomalies (syndactyly in the hand).
- Autosomal recessive condition.

Clinical features

- Most are asymptomatic.
- Diagnosis is an incidental finding.

Radiological features

- **CXR** – increased transradiancy of the affected hemithorax. Absence of the normal pectoralis soft tissue shadow.
- **CT** – confirms the absent muscle and normal lung.

Differential diagnosis

- Post mastectomy changes.
- Unilateral obliterative bronchiolites (e.g. Macleod's syndrome) may mimic Poland's syndrome.

Management

- No active management.

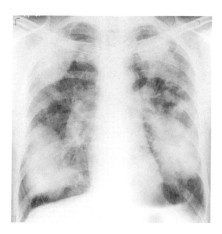

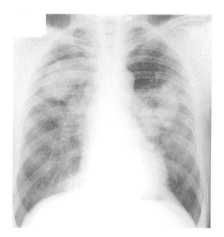
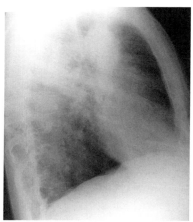

Progressive massive fibrosis – two cases. Large bilateral and symmetrical opacities at the periphery of the lung. Migration towards the hila. The medial border is often ill-defined with the lateral border sharp and parallel to the rib cage.

Differential diagnosis

- Sarcoid.
- Cryptogenic organising pneumonia.
- Lymphoma.
- Metastatic disease.

Management

- No active treatment available.

Pulmonary arterial hypertension

Characteristics

- Sustained pulmonary arterial pressure > 25 mmHg.
- Several causes
  - Excessive pulmonary blood flow, e.g. left to right shunts, AVMs and thyrotoxicosis.
  - Obliteration of pulmonary vasculature, e.g. pulmonary arterial emboli, idiopathic (primary pulmonary hypertension), vasculitis and chronic lung disease.
  - Excessive pulmonary vasoconstriction, e.g. hypoxia or drugs.
  - Secondary to pulmonary venous hypertension, e.g. left ventricular failure or mitral stenosis.
- Primary pulmonary hypertension is an idiopathic disease of young women.

Clinical features

- Can be asymptomatic, particularly early.
- Progressive SOB.
- Haemoptysis.
- Chest pains.
- Cyanosis.
- Hypoxia.
- Peripheral oedema.

Radiological features

- **CXR**
  - Enlargement of the main, right and left pulmonary arteries (main PA diameter >29 mm, right PA >16 mm and left PA >15 mm).
  - Rapid tapering of the pulmonary vasculature ('peripheral pruning').
  - The heart size may be normal or enlarged.
  - Look for underlying causes, e.g. chronic airways disease, AVMs or heart disease.
- **HRCT** – confirms pulmonary enlargement. There may be a mosaic pattern to the lungs with small-calibre vessels present in the low attenuation areas.
- **Echocardiography** – assessment of pressures within the pulmonary arterial system and looks for possible underlying causes.

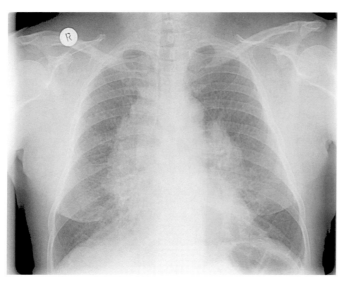

Sarcoidosis. '1-2-3 sign' – right paratracheal and right and left hilar nodes.

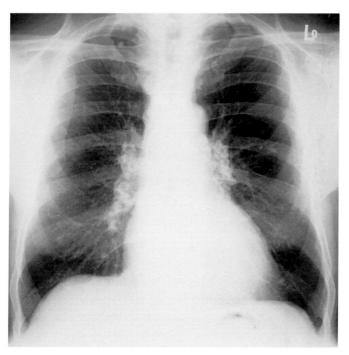

Sarcoidosis. Egg shell calcification of both hila.

the hilar are pulled superiorly and posteriorly. Lymph nodes can demonstrate egg shell calcification.
- **HRCT**
  - Very good at confirming irregular septal, bronchovascular and fissural nodularity. Traction bronchiectasis, fibrosis and ground glass change may be present. There may also be tracheobronchial stenosis. Also look for subdiaphragmatic, cardiac, bone, hepatic and splenic involvement on the same scan.

Differential diagnosis

- Lymphoma.
- Infection – TB.
- Lymphangitis carcinomatosis.
- Chronic hypersensitivity pneumonitis.

Management

- Biopsy or bronchoalveolar lavage may be necessary to gain histological confirmation, particularly as symptomatic cases may resemble active TB.
- Mainstay of treatment is steroids, which may be long term.

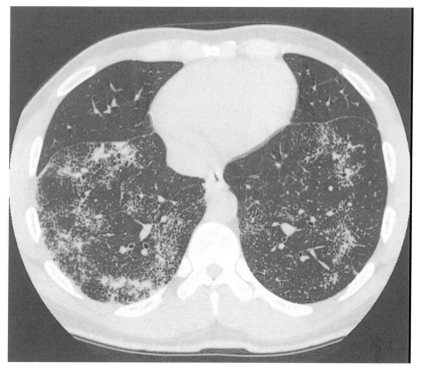

Sarcoidosis – HRCT. Irregular septal, bronchovascular and fissural nodularity.

Silicosis

Characteristics

- This is a specific pneumoconiosis caused by the inhalation of the inorganic dust particle silicone dioxide (mining, quarrying and sandblasting).
- The silica is phagocytosed by pulmonary macrophages. Cytotoxic reaction leads to the formation of non-caseating granulomata. These form small silicotic nodules. Pulmonary fibrosis develops as nodules coalesce.
- Acute and chronic forms.
  - The chronic form follows over 20 years of exposure.
  - The acute form may occur after as little as 1 year.
- Association with TB in 25%.
- Silicosis can develop into progressive massive fibrosis.

Clinical features

- May be asymptomatic.
- Non-productive cough.
- Dyspnoea – this is progressive.
- Weight loss, malaise.
- Hypoxia.
- Restrictive lung function.

Radiological features

- **CXR**
  - **Chronic form**: 3- to 10-mm nodules present in the upper and mid zones. Some of the nodules coalesce. There is hilar lymphadeno-pathy, some of which shows egg shell calcification. There may be upper lobe fibrotic change.
  - **Acute form**: bilateral lower lobe peripheral air space opacification and ground glass pattern.
  - **Progressive massive fibrosis**: masses (1 cm), usually in the poster-ior segment of the upper lobes, coalesce and are associated with hilar retraction. Cavitation may represent superimposed active TB infection.
- **HRCT**
  - Demonstrates small nodular opacities, interlobular septal thickening, fibrous parenchymal bands and ground glass pattern.

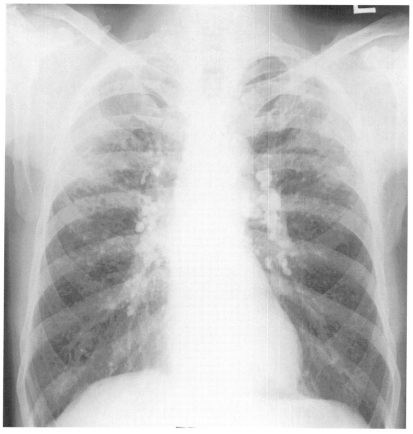

Silicosis. Egg shell calcification of both hila.

Differential diagnosis

- Sarcoidosis.
- TB.
- Miliary metastases.
- Other inhalational pneumoconiosis.

Management

- Unfortunately, despite removal of the causative dust, silicosis is often progressive.
- No active treatment available.

Subphrenic abscess

Characteristics

- Focal walled-off infected intra-abdominal collection lying in the sub-diaphragmatic space.
- Usually right sided.
- Gram-negative or anaerobic organisms are the usual pathogens.
- The source is usually from bowel (spread from diverticulitis, bowel infection/inflammation or even colonic malignancy).
- At increased risk are the elderly, immobile and immunosuppressed.

Clinical features

- Fever (can be swinging).
- Sweats.
- Weight loss.
- Malaise.
- Cough (diaphragmatic irritation).
- Dyspnoea.

Radiological features

- **CXR** – elevated hemidiaphragm. Pleural effusion (reactive). Subphrenic lucency or air-fluid level.
- **CT**
  - Wall enhancing sub-diaphragmatic collection.
  - May contain locules of air.
- The collection may breach the diaphragm and communicate with the pleural space.
- May be free intra-abdominal fluid.
- Look for bowel wall thickening or diverticulosis as a possible source of the sepsis.

Differential diagnosis

- Loculated pneumothorax.
- Lung abscess or empyema.
- Pneumoperitoneum.
- Interposed bowel, e.g. Chilaiditi's.
- Diaphragmatic eventration.
- Phrenic nerve palsy.

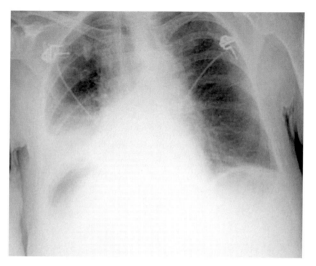

Subphrenic abscess. Note the large pocket of gas within a right subphrenic collection. This results in elevation of the right hemidiaphragm and a secondary right basal pleural effusion.

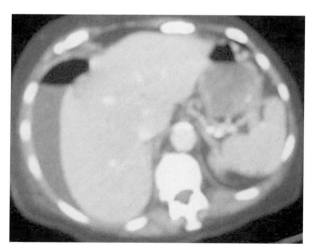

CT confirms the presence of gas within a right subphrenic collection.

Management

- Antibiotic therapy.
- Percutaneous drainage; may be US or CT guided.
- Occasionally surgical drainage is needed.
- Look for an underlying source of the infection. This is usually secondary to a primary bowel pathology – do in order not to miss a colonic malignancy.

Thoracoplasty

Characteristics

- Represents an old form of treatment for active TB infection.
- The principle involved deliberate and permanent collapse of the affected lung. TB organisms are obligate aerobes and the collapsed lung receives no oxygen, thus starving the infection.
- There are two main types of thoracoplasty.
  - Plombage – the placement of inert foreign bodies within the hemithorax collapsing the affected lung.
  - Rib excision with lung collapse.

Clinical features

- Many are asymptomatic.
- Complete unilateral thoracoplasty may be associated with dyspnoea or chest discomfort.

Radiological features

- **CXR**
  - **Plombage**
    - Radio-opaque or radiolucent well-circumscribed densities within the affected lung, usually the lung apex. The appearance often looks like 'ping pong balls'. Other inert substances may be used.
    - This may be associated with adjacent rib anomalies or absent ribs.
  - **Unilateral thoracoplasty**
    - Associated with more extensive rib anomalies/ rib excision.
    - The whole hemithorax is small with no significant aerated lung present.

Differential diagnosis

- Congenital anomalies including neurofibromatosis rarely resemble the appearances of thoracoplasty.

Management

- No active treatment required.

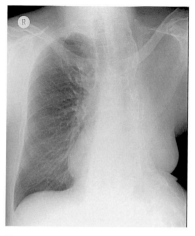

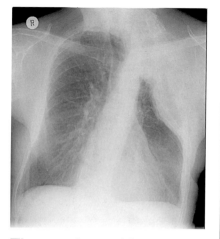

Thoracoplasty.

Thoracoplasty with plombage.

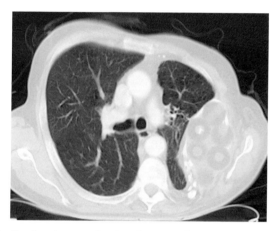

The lucite balls clearly seen in the thoracoplasty cavity.

Thymus – malignant thymoma

Characteristics

- Most common primary neoplasm of the anterior superior mediastinum.
- They are lymphoepithelial neoplasms and may be benign or malignant (30%).
- Demonstration of malignancy is based on behaviour rather than histological appearance.
- Presentation usually in middle age.
- Strong association with myasthenia gravis (35% of patients with a thymoma have myasthenia gravis).
- Other associations include red cell aplasia, hypogammaglobulinaemia and paraneoplastic syndromes.
- The malignant disease can spread to the mediastinum and pleura invading mediastinal and intrathoracic structures.

Clinical features

- Asymptomatic (50%) – incidentally picked up on CXR.
- Chest pains, dyspnoea, cough.
- Stridor, hoarse voice, dysphagia.
- SVC obstruction.
- Sweats, weight loss.
- Associated myasthenic symptoms.

Radiological features

- **CXR** – round/ovoid anterosuperior mediastinal mass (may be difficult to visualise). Widening of the mediastinum. Calcification may be present. Pleurally based metastatic masses may be present.
- **CT** – usually a homogeneous soft tissue mass in the anterior mediastinum with uniform enhancement. There may be cystic changes, patchy calcification and invasion of the mediastinal fat and other mediastinal structures. Pleural metastatic soft tissue masses may be present.
- **MRI** – similar appearances and findings to CT. However, it may allow clearer demonstration of soft tissue invasion.

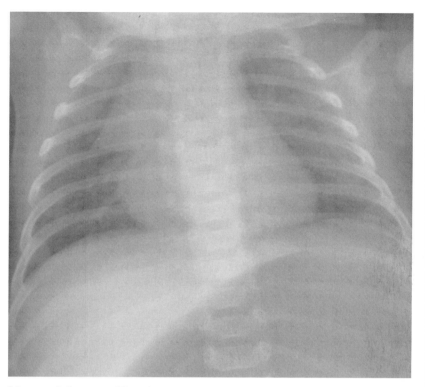

Normal thymus. This demonstrates the classical **'sail-sign'** of normal thymic tissue in a neonate. The normal thymus usually undergoes complete atrophy by adolescence.

Tuberculosis

Characteristics

- *Mycobacterium tuberculosis* (TB) is an aerobic bacillus.
- High cause of morbidity and mortality worldwide.
- Rising incidence due to increasing susceptibility and antibiotic resistance.
- Susceptible groups include immunocompromised, elderly, alcoholics and immigrants from third world countries.
- TB predominately affects the lungs but spread via lymphatics and blood vessels allows dissemination to other organs (pericardium, gastrointestinal and genitourinary tracts, bone and the CNS).
- Diagnosis may sometimes be difficult – direct sputum/tissue microscopy or culture. Immunological skin testing using Heaf or Mantoux tests. Unfortunately the patient needs to be able to host an immune response to aid diagnosis. In some patients this response is absent due to immunosuppression.
- Three main types of pulmonary tuberculous infection:
  - Primary.
  - Post primary or reactivation.
  - Miliary.
- A tuberculoma represents a focal mass lesion of uncertain tuberculous infective activity.

Clinical features

- Cough, SOB, sputum or haemoptysis.
- Weight loss, fatigue and malaise.
- Pyrexia and night sweats.
- Progressive, rapid and debilitating symptoms suggest miliary spread of the infection.
- Always consider the diagnosis in at–risk groups and patients who fail to respond to standard antibiotic regimes.

Radiological features

- **CXR**
  - **Primary**
    - May be active or inactive infection.
    - Scarring and calcification (lung and lymph nodes) suggest inactive disease.

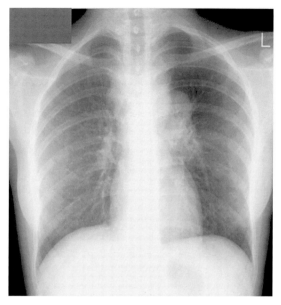

Primary TB. Right paratracheal and left hilar adenopathy.

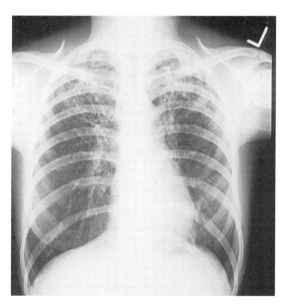

Post primary TB. Linear parenchymal streaking extending into both apices, with associated retraction of both hila. The findings are of bilateral upper lobe fibrosis.

- Consolidation, small focal nodularity, lymphadenopathy and effusions suggest active infection.
- A Ghon focus is a peripheral area of lung consolidation.
- **Post primary**
  - Again may be active or inactive.
  - Focal scarring and lung distortion ± cavitation. Usually in upper lobes.
  - Adenopathy and effusions are much less common.
  - Fungal infections may develop in active cavities (myecetomas).
- **Miliary infection**
  - Multiple small discrete widespread pulmonary nodules.
- **Reactivation of TB** can be difficult to diagnose. Comparison with old films for changes in appearance is helpful. Increased soft tissue and cavitation suggest active infection.
- **CT** and **HRCT** – demonstrate occult soft tissue masses, cavitation and lymphadenopathy. Other features include reticulonodular change and 'tree-in-bud' appearances in keeping with endobronchial disease. The lymph nodes are characteristically necrotic on contrast-enhanced studies.

Differential diagnosis

- Other infections including non *Tuberculosis mycobacterium*.
- Lymphoma.
- Sarcoid.
- Miliary metastases may mimic miliary TB disease.

Management

- Current treatment is 6–12 months of a quadruple antibiotic regime.
- Patient contacts should be screened for active disease and treated where appropriate.
- Always consider reactivation of TB in susceptible groups, and symptomatic patients previously exposed to TB.

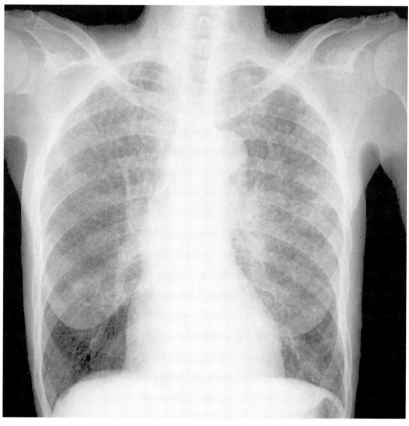

Miliary TB. Multiple tiny nodules scattered throughout both lungs.

Varicella pneumonia

Characteristics

- Usually presents in adults.
- Severe chest infection which may require hospitalisation.
- Vesicular rash and patchy diffuse lung changes.
- The pneumonia can heal with tiny calcified granulomata throughout the lungs. These have a characteristic appearance on CXR and should be recognised and not confused with alternative diagnoses.

Clinical features

- Acute infection – cough, sputum, fever, malaise, dyspnoea and vesicular rash.
- Post infection – asymptomatic.

Radiological features

- **CXR**
  - Acute infection – patchy, diffuse consolidation often coalescing at the bases and hila. Lung nodules may be present in 30%.
  - Post infection – tiny discrete calcified granulomata throughout the lungs.

Differential diagnosis

- Acutely – any bacterial or fungal pneumonia.
- Post infection – the appearances may rarely mimic miliary TB or calcified metastases (e.g. thyroid). Clinical correlation is diagnostic.

Management

- Acute infection
  - ABC.
  - Oxygen.
  - May require antiviral therapy and occasionally steroids.
  - May require ventilatory support.
- Post infection
  - No active management.

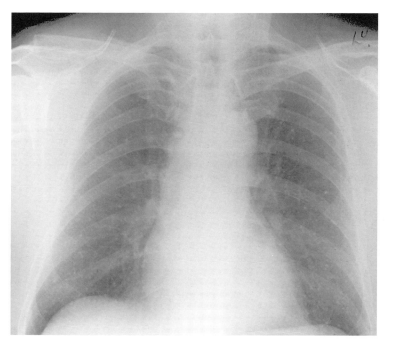

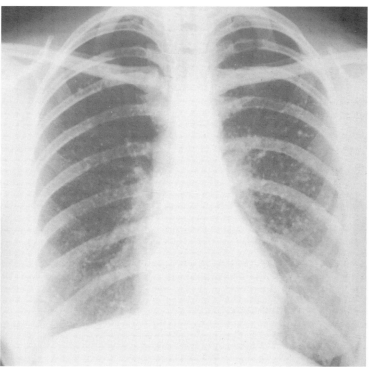

Previous varicella pneumonia – two cases. Multiple calcified nodules scattered throughout both lungs.

Wegener's granulomatosis

Characteristics

- This is a multisystem disease of unknown aetiology.
- Characterised by necrotising vasculitis of medium and small-sized vessels, tissue necrosis (which may be granulomatous) and inflammation which is both acute and chronic.
- Classically involves the lungs (95%), kidneys (85% – glomerulonephritis) and paranasal sinuses (90%).
- Other organs can be involved (eyes, skin, joints, CNS, GI tract and heart).
- M > F 2:1.
- Presents in childhood or old age (70s).
- c-ANCA positive (96% sensitive). Beware active TB infection, which can cause mild serum elevation of this antibody, sometimes making diagnosis difficult.

Clinical features

- Variable presentation
- Stridor (tracheal inflammation).
- Cough, haemoptysis.
- SOB, fever, chest pain.
- Sinus pain and purulent sputum.
- Epistaxis, saddle-shaped nose (destruction of the nasal cartilage).
- Joint pains.
- Weight loss, abdominal pains, diarrhoea.
- Cutaneous rash and nodules.
- Proptosis.
- Peripheral and central neuropathies.

Radiological features

- **CXR** – pulmonary nodules of varying size. They can cavitate and can occur anywhere in the lung. Patchy, sometimes extensive consolidation or ground glass change (which may reflect pulmonary haemorrhage). Pleural effusions in one-third.
- **CT** – confirms **CXR** appearances. The nodules may have a rim of ground glass around them (halo sign secondary to infarction). In addition there may be peripheral pleurally based wedge shaped infarcts. There may also be tracheobronchial narrowing due to inflammation. Lymphadenopathy is not a feature.

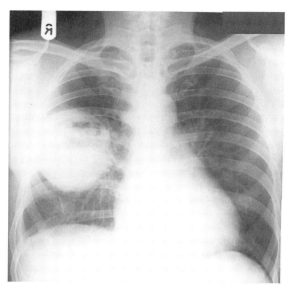

Wegner's granulomatosis. Large cavitating lung mass in the right mid zone.

Differential diagnosis

- Churg–Strauss syndrome – this is asthma associated with a small vessel vasculitis, p-ANCA positive.
- Rheumatoid arthritis (RA) – some forms of RA can mimic Wegener's granulomatosis.
- Infection – particularly fungal infections, TB or septic emboli from disseminated infection.
- Cryptogenic organising pneumonia.
- Metastatic disease.

Management

- Treatment with corticosteroids.
- Long-term therapy with cytotoxic drugs (e.g. cyclophosphamide).
- Renal disease may lead to renal failure requiring dialysis and ultimately consideration for renal transplantation.

Westermark's sign

Characteristics

- This represents a focal area of oligaemia usually due to a distal pulmonary embolus. It is seen in 5% of pulmonary embolic patients.
- Rarer causes including tumour compression and inflammatory vasculitis can produce similar radiographic appearances.

Clinical features

- SOB.
- Cough, haemoptysis.
- Pleuritic chest pain.
- Deep leg vein thrombus.
- Hypoxia.
- Hypotension.
- Collapse.

Radiological features

- **CXR** – wedge shaped area of low attenuation
  - Other radiographic features of pulmonary embolic disease include:
    - Fleischner's sign – local widening of pulmonary artery due to distension from clot.
    - Hampton's hump - segmental pleurally based wedge shaped opacity representing a pulmonary infarct.
- **CT** (**CTPA**) – Filling defects within the pulmonary arteries.

Differential diagnosis

- Occasionally focal areas of apparent lucency are demonstrated in areas adjacent to pulmonary consolidation or "ground glass" change. These areas of increased attenuation may represent infection, fluid or pulmonary haemorrhage and are abnormal. The apparent lucent area is spared lung and actually represents the normal lung.

Management

- ABC.
- Oxygen.
- Anticoagulation if PE is confirmed.

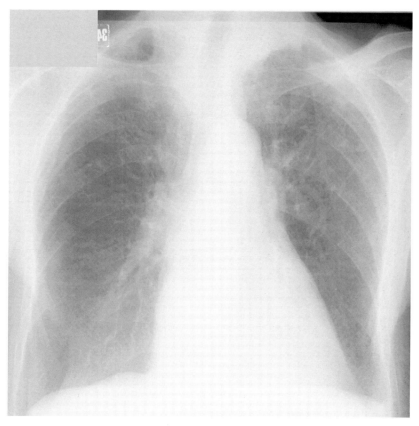

Westermark sign – Pulmonary embolus. A large part of the right hemithorax is hypodense due to oligaemia, secondary to vasoconstriction distal to an embolus